COLPOSCOPY AND CERVICAL PATHOLOGY

Edited by **Rajamanickam Rajkumar**

Colposcopy and Cervical Pathology
http://dx.doi.org/10.5772/65158
Edited by Rajamanickam Rajkumar

Contributors

Marta García -Yuste, Ana Muñoz Ledesma, Mayte Navarro Monge, Ovidiu Balacescu, Loreadana Balacescu, Oana Tudoran, Patriciu Achimas, Oana Baldasici, Codrina Ancuta, Eugen Ancuta, Dumitru Sofroni, Angelica Judith Granados López, Jesús Adrián López, Hiroyuki Kuramoto, Toshiko Jobo, Rajamanickam Rajkumar

Published by InTech

Janeza Trdine 9, 51000 Rijeka, Croatia

Publishing Process Manager Nina Kalinic
Technical Editor SPi Global
Cover InTech Design team

First published October, 2017
Printed in Croatia
Legal deposit, Croatia: National and University Library in Zagreb

Additional hard copies can be obtained from orders@intechopen.com

Colposcopy and Cervical Pathology , Edited by Rajamanickam Rajkumar
p. cm.
Print ISBN 978-953-51-3537-1
Online ISBN 978-953-51-3538-8

For EU product safety concerns:
IN TECH d.o.o., Prolaz Marije Krucifikse Kozulić 3, 51000 Rijeka, Croatia,
info@intechopen.com or visit our website at intechopen.com.

Meet the editor

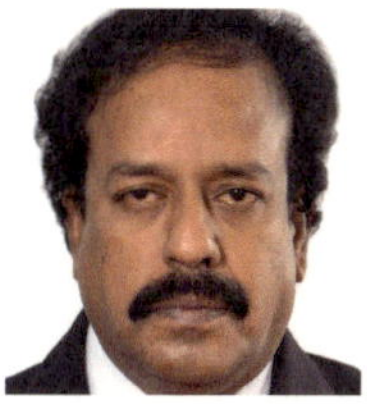

Rajamanickam Rajkumar, professor of Community Medicine and PhD guide at Meenakshi Medical College, Kanchipuram, Tamil Nadu, India, was inspired at school age to become a doctor by his mother Navamani, a teacher, supported by Christine Matthews, an Irish missionary, working at Christian Medical College, Vellore. He won a meritorious gold medal for his research on leprosy eradication in India, during his MD, which he passed with distinction in 1993. Due to his love to serve for rural people, he worked at the Christian Fellowship Community Health Centre, Ambillikai, Tamil Nadu, greatly influenced by Padmabushan Dr. Jacob Cherian. Burdened by the large number of cervical cancer cases attending this small rural hospital, Raj wrote to the IARC/WHO for guidance, in prevention and control of cervical cancer. With IARC, he initiated a Rural Population-Based Cancer Registry in 1996. He was honored with his PhD degree from Open University of Colombo for this pioneer work. He received training in colposcopy and precancer management in the UK, Ireland, and Singapore. In 2001, he implemented a large-scale screening program, using the village-level health workers/nurses and VIA screening technology. This project of IARC was a great success. In 2011, in collaboration with the Society for Colposcopy and Cervical Pathology, Singapore, and The Ohio State University Medical Center, USA, he formed a society for training doctors and nurses in cervical cancer prevention. In 2012, he received the "Best Teacher and Research Award" from Meenakshi Academy of Higher Education and Research (MAHER), Chennai, India.

In 2016, he formed a network of medical and nursing colleges to undertake cervical cancer and HPV screening programs among the most underserved and unreached poor women of rural India. Currently, he is involved in primordial prevention of HPV and guiding PhD research, in cancer prevention, at national and international universities. He invites international collaborations in cervical cancer prevention and HPV vaccines and research.

Contents

Preface

Cervical cancer screening programs, worldwide, apply the first-level screening tests like VIA and cytology, for identifying early lesions of the cervical intraepithelial neoplasia (CIN). On the basis of these results, women are referred for colposcopy, which identifies the topographical characteristics of CIN, and directed biopsy is performed for confirmative diagnosis. The specimen is sent to pathology laboratory where cervical pathology experts make a histological diagnosis of CIN. Based on this, the woman is called for precancer treatment with modalities like cryotherapy, loop electrosurgical excision procedure (LEEP), cold coagulation, and laser ablation. Once the precancer lesion is ablated, the woman is followed for a period of about 3 years with periodical histopathology examinations. After this, she is declared free of disease status, and she is not having the possibilities of developing cervical cancer.

This universal protocol ensures high success rate of cervical cancer screening programs. But if the woman who are referred for colposcopy does not comply, due to many reasons like fear, anxiety, and socioeconomic and cultural factors, the efforts made by screening programs will not be successful. The underutilization of services results in wastage of resources.

To improve resource effectiveness, empowerment of women is advocated. The entire system of cervical cancer screening should start from teenage girls with primordial prevention of HPV infections, by education and vaccination. Primary prevention is the next level with early diagnosis and treatment of precancer lesions. At this level, the woman is saved from cervical cancer, which is the purpose of the screening.

Change in behavior by education and empowerment of individuals, families, and communities is the key to success. This book is a masterpiece with international authors contributing from their rich clinical experience. The editor adds value by his experiences at community level, during successful implementation of one of the largest cervical cancer screening programs in developing countries. The InTech publishers would achieve their goal if the readers are inspired to transfer technologies and translate research for preventing cervical cancer, especially in developing countries, with limited resources.

Our mission is Inspired to Inspire and Lighted to Lighten.

Wishing the readers a pleasurable and purposeful reading!

Dr. Rajamanickam Rajkumar, MD, PhD
Professor, Community Medicine
Meenakshi Medical College Hospital & Research Institute
Constitute of MAHER, Kanchipuram
Tamil Nadu, India

Section 1

Introduction

Chapter 1

Introductory Chapter: Colposcopy and Cervical Pathology in Cervical Cancer Screening Programs: Resource Effectiveness, Concepts, and Models of "Raj"©

Rajamanickam Rajkumar

Additional information is available at the end of the chapter

http://dx.doi.org/10.5772/intechopen.69692

1. Introduction

The author is pleased to share his experiences, the concepts, and models he evolved, during his role as the Principal Investigator of large-scale, cervical cancer screening programs, and Human Papillomavirus—HPV prevalence studies, in Tamil Nadu, India, during early 2000.

The resources available in any setting, region, community, and country need prudent management. Cost effectiveness and cost benefit are important strategies in health economics. Improving on these, the author introduces a strategy "Resource Effectiveness," to be considered by the healthcare systems in general and healthcare planners in particular.

The research articles in this book, constructively contribute to the globally important topic "Colposcopy and Cervical Pathology," especially in the context of cervical cancer screening programs, in low and limited resource settings. The two important services are yet to be planned for ideal use and optimum benefit. "Poverty in Abundance" situations are not uncommon. The author is pleased to make efforts for both ends to meet. The philosophy of "Lighted to Lighten" is applied for the beneficiary community and health system research. Sparking strategies, current concepts, and modifiable models are presented for the benefit of science globally and society worldwide.

I am greatly privileged to be the editor and also write this introductory review chapter as one of the team members to enrich and support the noble efforts of the INTECH publishers and esteemed authors. The concepts and models, recommended here, are to be appropriated to suit individual situations, but the objective of this endeavor is to achieve the targets set by the "Cervical cancer prevention programs" in all settings, universally.

2. Concept 1: "RAM of RAJ for Resource effectiveness"

The resources as conceived by the experience of the author are classified as **T12** and means of achieving effectiveness for each resource input is explained. This model is called Resource Appropriate Management—**RAM of Raj**.

2.1. Resource appropriate management

(1)	Time	Single visit approach
(2)	Talent	Create local manpower
(3)	Team	Community health volunteers
(4)	Treasure	Community/self-supported
(5)	Technique	Integrated with available primary health care
(6)	Technology	Simple, affordable, e.g., via portable Colposcope cryotherapy—cold coagulation Affordable, acceptable, available
(7)	Technologist	Out sourcing contracts, part timers, volunteers from existing government hospitals, medical schools, and private and medical institutions
(8)	Technology transfer	Hemostats like silver nitrate crystals can be used instead of Monsel's paste, which is expensive and not available in many countries, during LEEP/LLETZ
(9)	Trainings at home	Training programs at project sites and not abroad
(10)	Training places	Local establishment and in medical schools, government hospitals, E-learning
(11)	Translational research	Global health researches for inputs and research collaboration with local medical institutions
(12)	Task and talk	Advocacy and fund raising

3. Concept 2: "RISES" model of RAJ—for effective screening

Cervical cancer prevention—by Raj's "RISES" model.

3.1. Raj's interactive squares for effective screening—RISES model

The prevention strategies for cervical cancer are based on four levels and three stages, for all the intervention principles.

The four levels are as follows:

1. Primordial prevention
2. Primary prevention
3. Secondary prevention
4. Tertiary prevention

The three stages are as follows:

1. Individual stage
2. Family stage
3. Community stage

The interactions of these are presented in the 16-square table below.

		Stage 1	Stage 2	Stage 3
		Individual	**Family**	**Community**
Level 1	Primordial prevention Objective: Prevention of risk factors	Teenage girls—education about HPV infections and need for HPV vaccination	Education about HPV to all women in the household Condom use as a preventive measure for HPV transmission HPV vaccination for eligible women Participation in HPV/CaCx screening programs	Schools—education to teenage girls about menstrual hygiene, sexual hygiene Protection with HPV vaccination for eligible girls Plan and implement HPV/CaCx screening programs
Level 2	Primary prevention Objectives: Health promotion specific protection	To attend HPV/Ca Cx screening programs Compliance for colposcopy referrals. Diagnosis by cytology/biopsy and have evidence of disease status. Regular follow up and treatment—understand the importance of cervical pathology services	All eligible women to be motivated to attend HPV/Ca Cx screening programs Compliance for colposcopy referrals. Diagnosis by cytology/biopsy and have evidence of disease status. Regular follow up and treatment	To plan, implement screening programs - All eligible women to be motivated to attend HPV/Ca Cx screening programs Compliance for colposcopy referrals—encouraged and enhanced by community healthcare volunteers. Diagnosis by cytology/biopsy and have evidence of disease status. Regular follow up and treatment—encouraged and ensured by volunteers

		Stage 1	Stage 2	Stage 3
		Individual	Family	Community
Level 3	Secondary prevention Objectives: Early diagnosis and treatment of Cx Ca precursors	Self-empowerment for: Compliance in colposcopy referrals. Diagnosis by cytology/ biopsy and have evidence of disease status. To have regular follow up and treatment	Family empowerment for compliance in colposcopy referrals. Diagnosis by cytology/ biopsy and have evidence of disease status. To have regular follow up and treatment	Community empowerment for compliance in colposcopy referrals. Diagnosis by cytology/ biopsy and have evidence of disease status. To have regular follow up and treatment
Level 4	Tertiary prevention Disability Limitation and Rehabilitation	Being self-empowered to undergo colposcopy examinations cytology/ biopsy diagnostic procedures. Understand and accept the diagnosis. To have treatment done for diseases status—CaCx precursor stages. Compliance for regular follow-up services to attain disease cure status	Family empowered to undergo colposcopy examinations cytology/ biopsy diagnostic procedures. Understand and accept the diagnosis. To have treatment done for diseases status–CaCx precursor stages. compliance for regular follow-up services to attain disease cure status	Community empowered and program assurance colposcopy examinations cytology/ biopsy diagnostic procedures. Understand and accept the diagnosis. To have treatment done for diseases status—CaCx precursor stages. Compliance for regular follow-up services to attain disease cure status

3.2. RAJ's interactive squares for effective screening: RISES concept

This concept is diagrammatically represented in the above model—RISES.

The "RISES" concept is elaborative discussion about the strategies to be considered in HPV/ cervical cancer screening and treatment programs for improving community compliance for all the services of the program, especially for colposcopy referrals and precancer treatments. The HPV vaccination programs also can follow the concepts with tailored modifications.

The evaluation/cost-effective and cost benefit analysis should be aimed at reaching "Resource Effectiveness," which could be the objective of the "Health Economy" of the program.

4. Interventions should start with teenage girls at school/community levels

It is very appropriate to start or plan for an HPV screening program for girls in their 12 years onward, from the school life. Menstrual hygiene and sexual hygiene lessons to be taught with planned, defined, focused, valid, and reliable syllabus. The lessons should be well prepared by the health service providers and the messenger, message, media, and effectiveness should be tailored according to the receivers and the micro/macroenvironment. Sanitary napkins may be provided by the healthcare system.

The use of male condoms is much advocated for its many benefits, such as birth control and prevention of transmission of sexual diseases, including HPV transmission.

HPV vaccination should be included as a private/public practice or policy. The efficacy of HPV vaccination should be assessed initially, concurrently, and periodically. Policies should be formulated and implemented by the local authorities.

Screening programs for HPV/cervical cancer, in many situations, face the problem of low compliance. Empowerment through education, socioeconomic inputs, and appropriate, affordable, acceptable, available healthcare services are important components to enhance compliance.

5. Concept 3: "RAIN-REACH" concept of RAJ for effective health education: health education

5.1. The RAIN–REACH concept of Raj

The RAIN criteria for health education are enlisted below:

(1) R = Reliability

(2) A = Adequacy

(3) I = Innovative

(4) N = Need–RAIN

5.1.1. R = Reliability

The reliability is for

- The health education message
- The health educator
- The health education system

5.1.1.1. Health education message

The "Message" should always be tailor made. The language should be local, simple, understandable, and supported by figures/photos/diagrams for the uneducated population. The use of complicated vocabulary, slogans, and jargons should be avoided. The message should be taint free of race/religion/caste/creed/ethnicity/politics. The use of scary and frightening messages, photos of advanced cancer stages of patients, photos of complicated surgeries, and medical instruments/procedures should be avoided. Pessimistic and negative statements should be avoided. It is very effective to have messages with positive attitude and pleasantness.

5.1.1.2. Health educator

The community is very receptive to people of their own identities. The educator should be taking into account the local beliefs, cultures, and custom. It is good to train "Local Health Volunteers –LHVs" to deliver the messages. The education should be an ongoing process and so it is suggested that the educators are from the community, of the community, and by the community. They should be living locally and thus ensure all time accessibility for the community for clarifications and explanations. This role of educator also involves counseling, especially in situations where one has to reveal the diagnosis and advice for further investigations like colposcopy and cervical pathology, from the hospitals. Thus, reliability of the educator helps in compliance.

5.1.1.3. The health education system

The cervical cancer screening programs, colposcopy, and cervical pathology services should be planned in such a way that they are integrated services of an ongoing healthcare system. In some countries, it is called the "Primary Health Care" system. Holistic care models are more effective and successful than "Organ specific health care services." The healthcare system, which has addressed many health problems of morbidity, mortality, maternal outcomes, and control and prevention of communicable and noncommunicable diseases, provides an ideal platform, well-equipped and empowered, to take up the challenges faced in cervical cancer screening programs and the components of colposcopy and cervical pathology, thus ensuring success in achieving the goals of the programs.

5.1.2. A = Adequacy/appropriateness

The health education message should be adequate, starting from a normal stage to abnormal stage, explaining the gradual transition of the disease process, its reversibility and interventions/cure at each stage, as decided by the health education receiver. The message should not be depicting the advanced cancer stage clinical photos. Instead, details of the normal cervix, inflammations and treatment, changes in precancer stages and treatment, importance of colposcopy and cervical pathology services, the accessibility and affordability should be well explained and clarifications offered wherever needed.

5.1.3. I = Innovativeness

The people are more receptive to innovative and interesting messages which may stimulate them for action. For example, 10 tips for cervical health, top 10 screening and treatment methods for healthy cervix, and top 10 risk factors to be avoided for womb's welfare can be used. It is advisable, not to use the word "cancer, no cure, but death" in the messages. The author has tried using a teaching model—whole apple fruit given to the woman. Each receives an apple and she keeps it in hand. We ask them to draw a small circle at one end of the apple and paint it white using crayons. It is explained that the apple is their uterus and the small circle they have painted white is the acetowhite area seen on their ectocervix on visual inspection after applying acetic acid, similar to the paint they have used. This is also the picture seen in colposcopy with a magnified image. We tell them that there is nothing to worry but we take a small punch for cervical pathology, a bit of tissue taken for examination. They are also told to scrap a piece from the white area in their apple and we explain that it is called biopsy in medical terms. Then we lead them for further actions. We ask the whether they will throw away the full apple because of the white area or scrap away the white area and retain the whole apple. The usual answer is that they will retain the apple. In the same way, it is explained that their acetowhite area will be removed by cryotherapy/cryo-coagulation/laser ablation or loop electro excision procedure—LEEP, and the uterus is retained. The women get convinced. The health educators shall plan such innovativeness for their programs.

5.1.4. N = Need

The "felt need" of time/place/person. The providers of health education should take into consideration, the need of their program, in the context of time/place/person.

5.1.4.1. Time

The convenience of the beneficiaries should be kept in mind rather than the official working time of the program workers. It is suggested that the education programs can be conducted in the community during late evenings, when people are back from their work and are having time for education sessions. Appointments also can be fixed with individuals for health education slots.

5.1.4.2. Place

One may be surprised to find that very sensitive and personal messages are conveyed in public places. The health planners may have the idea that more people would see their messages displayed in public places like market, bus station, and other public gathering places. But to convey private issues like cervical cancer/breast cancer screening, the appropriate place would be in the privacy of the homes. This sort of precautions for privacy and confidentiality should be considered, especially in conservative communities.

5.1.4.3. Person

The methods such as child to parent education, satisfied customers' word of mouth, and peer group education are successful strategies. Men to men and women to women education are also to be practiced in certain situations. Barriers of communication need to be kept in mind in gender-related education. We have discussed the RAIN concept for education to be successful, which is strategic approach for the healthcare providers.

6. "REACH" concept for healthcare beneficiaries

R = Reception/retain/recall/respond/react/recommend—R6, E = Effectiveness, A = Acceptability, C = Change in behavior, H = Health target achievement—REACH

6.1. The R6

6.1.1. Reception

The health education messages should be positive, pleasant, palatable, and practicable for the community, and the messages should not be frightening, scary, negative like telling about an advanced stage of cancer and how many deaths occur and likewise. Pleasant communication is the key for good reception.

6.1.2. Retain

Repeated messages and reproducible facts help the community to retain the essentials of what has been communicated. The strategy of "indoctrination" plays a major role for retention of the messages in the minds of healthcare beneficiaries.

6.1.3. Recall/respond/react

These are the links in the behavior change process and these depend on small group discussions, interactive teaching, and learning sessions.

6.1.4. Recommend

The best way of education in health programs would be by word of mouth from the satisfied customers. The ultimate goal that can be achieved in screening programs would be compliance and recommendation to other potential beneficiaries.

6.2. E = Effectiveness

The effectiveness of education in cervical cancer screening programs can be measured objectively by assessing the change in knowledge-attitude-practice, about the subject that has been focused during the education process. An increased level of knowledge leads to change in the attitude. But for the desired action to be achieved, there should be constant motivation by various means and methods. For example, a woman who never knew the benefits of cervical screening now understands the importance and offers herself for the screening tests.

6.3. A = Acceptability

The woman, who has been well educated and motivated, are now at the screening clinic. It is very important for the health planners to provide her "acceptability" at every stage of process and procedure. Providing all services under one roof is a good strategy. Services offered free of cost, at discounts, with incentives, cost benefit of the diagnosis, and treatment services like the colposcopy, cervical pathology, and precancer treatment modalities should be well explained to the beneficiary at the initial entry level and at all other stages and instant clarifications of doubts, allay of fear, should be done, which largely comforts the women and greatly help in cooperation and compliance.

6.4. C = Change in behavior

The desired change in behavior of the healthcare beneficiaries is the expected goal of all the education programs. It is more important in cervical cancer screening programs. An individual who was illiterate, ignorant about cervical health is being educated, motivated and she accepts screening, understands her initial results. Then, she is referred for colposcopy if her primary tests like VIA/VILI/Pap smear results indicate a precancer condition. Those who are apprehensive, hostile, uncooperative, and noncompliant are now having a change in behavior and respond positively. The women subject themselves for colposcopy examinations and biopsy and treatment procedures. Effecting this change is the mark of success of the cervical screening programs.

6.5. H = Health for all

All the deliberations so far would eventually help in the process of attaining a level of health, which is socioeconomically productive for the individual. Attainment of this level of health, by the individual, leads to attainment at family level, community, and country level. This is the achievement of the goal "Health for all," as envisioned by the World Health Organization (WHO).

7. Conclusion

Colposcopy and cervical pathology services, in screening programs, worldwide, are highly resource intensive. The resources which the author considers are as follows:

Time, talent, team, treasure, techniques, technology, technologists, transfer of technology, teaching and training sources, translational efforts and research, task and talk—the **T 12**.

Health management systems across the world need to plan for resource effective strategies for colposcopy and cervical pathology in cervical cancer screening programs, which are currently highly resource intensive components. In this chapter, the author has discussed about **REACT, RISES,** and **RAIN-REACH concepts of RAJ**. Hope that the publishers, readers, healthcare planners, healthcare providers, and most importantly the people are richly benefitted, and the united contribution pays its dividends.

Acknowledgements

The author gratefully acknowledges the intellectual intimacy and boundless love of Rixon Raj and Rijula Raj in perception and delivery of the concepts and models in this chapter.

Author details

Rajamanickam Rajkumar

Address all correspondence to: rajcfchc@gmail.com

Community Medicine, Meenakshi Medical College Hospital and Research Institute, Meenakshi Academy of Higher Education and Research—MAHER, Kanchipuram, Tamil Nadu, India

Section 2

Colposcopy

Chapter 2

Psychosocial Aspects of Colposcopic Assessment: Perspectives and Strategies for Physicians

Eugen Ancuta, Dumitru Sofroni, Codrina Ancuta, Larisa Sofroni, Ion Mereuta, Lilian Gutu and Emil Anton

Additional information is available at the end of the chapter

http://dx.doi.org/10.5772/intechopen.69160

Abstract

The purpose of this work is to determine perspectives, misconceptions, psychology adjustments and useful strategies of women living with dilemmas about their malignant lesions which can be detected through the colposcopy. Colposcopic assessment following abnormal Pap test has resulted in a long list of concerns: fear of having cancer, periodic obligations related to follow-up, balancing treatment of premalignant disease with quality of life, pain or discomfort and long-term impact on their families or limited social support. How prepared are they to adapt to their diagnosis? New diagnosis results in patient not being able to listen well or to understand her medical situation. The success of the outcome and procedure takes time to deduce the concerns she has regarding her diagnosis, treatment and appropriate follow-up. Several physicians endorse a wide range of barriers with respect to diagnosis and management of the disease: organizational or patient issues. Furthermore, patient appears to be important for the effective treatment than to identify and assess psychosocial problems among women diagnosed with cancer. In conclusion, physician provides effective treatment, but fails to address psychosocial issues associated with the illness. It is necessary to define the condition more clearly by studying patients and their psychosocial problems.

Keywords: colposcopy, cancer patients, psychosocial

1. Introduction

The purpose of this work is to determine perspectives, misconceptions, psychology adjustments and useful strategies of women living with dilemmas about their premalignant or malignant lesions which can be detected through colposcopy.

In the last few decades, there has been growing interest in the field of psychosocial aspects on women diagnosed with cancer or severe dysplasia.

Approximately 10 million United States cancer patients require appropriate psychosocial interventions and support programmes [1].

Psychological impact of cancer is a universal phenomenon, but the caring concept varies among different countries and cultures. Thus, the physician-patient relationship forms the basis of what constitutes caring for the patient [2–4].

Psychosocial aspects are directed by the idea that psychosocial issues are integrated into the overall management and treatment of the disease [5].

Psychological reaction to their disease has become a challenge for the oncologist in the second part of the twentieth century.

Some of the patients will develop psychiatric disorders such as anxiety, depression and adjustment disorders [2, 6, 7].

Having cancer can affect the brain and cause discomfort to the patients or may change their relationship with family, friends or colleagues [3].

Unfortunately, the achievements in providing care for the women diagnosed with cancer have not been correlated by remarkable advances in providing care for psychological symptoms and social consequences of cancer [2, 3].

Health policymakers, researchers or health insurers should respond to the psychosocial aspects of cancer patients. Cancer leaves patients with nonreversible consequences and requires long period of care [3].

2. Objectives

As the entire cancer trajectory including follow -up care to survivorship, emotional, spiritual and cultural issues, family support including social needs, child assistance, financial assistance and their potential applications to our context (must be a part of supportive cancer care) has multiple dimensions, we elected to focus on the psychosocial aspects of cancer survivors [2, 3].

Also, the subject has multiple dimensions; thus, we choose to focus on psychosocial aspects for cancer patients and their potential applications to my country. The goals of supportive care experts are to identify psychological repercussions of cancer diagnosis including concerns about body image, about sexuality or fertility, discrimination, fear of relapse, family's support, maintaining their own employment or being re-assimilated by their colleagues or friends [2].

The objectives have been focused on how to integrate the psychosocial aspects of terminal illness into supportive care from the time of diagnosis toward the end of the patient's life.

3. Rebuilding psychosocial care for cancer patients diagnosed after colposcopy-guided biopsy: gathering information

Many women diagnosed with cancer can be managed as a chronic disease [3, 6].

Physical examination, vital signs, gynaecological examination, Pap test, biopsy and laboratory values such as haematology, chemistry, urinalysis and histological evaluation were used for cancer diagnosis.

The findings can be accepted and should be interpreted with caution.

In the last few decades, there has been growing interest in the field of psychosocial aspects on women diagnosed with cancer or severe dysplasia by colposcopic examination. Because diagnostic and treatment of cancer have been associated with a higher risk of severe depression, it is important to evaluate the relationship between gynaecologists and their patients in order to improve communication skills and to identify any clinically relevant abnormal findings [2, 3].

Women with abnormal cervical cytology are at a great risk of developing cervical cancer.

Persistent HPV infection is necessary for the development of cervical cancer.

To facilitate the best possible care for women with abnormal Pap test, colposcopy is performed. For women with abnormal cytology results, colposcopic examinations have the advantage of prompt diagnosis. A colposcope is used to indicate and evaluate the presence of precancerous or cancerous lesions. After examination, the physician may obtain for directed biopsies from abnormal areas.

In Romania, National Cervical Screening Program is associated with a reduction in the incidence of invasive cervical cancer. This program is safe, effective, efficient and based on evidence.

Women colposcopic assessment following an abnormal Pap test has resulted in a long list of concerns: fear of having cancer, periodic obligations related to follow-up, balancing treatment of premalignant disease with quality of life, concern about pain or discomfort and long-term impact on their families or limited social support [3, 8].

How prepared are they to adapt to their diagnosis?

An abnormal cytology result can cause alteration in understanding the recommendations they receive and types of reactions. It may be helpful to provide information about medical procedures in order to maintain the balance of the physician-patient conversation.

The damage caused by hormone therapy, radiotherapy or chemotherapy often leads to functional disabilities or limitations in activities of daily living or capacity for work. Physical symptoms interfere with their mental functions. Despite the administration of analgesics , the pain is not eliminated and the distress of living with physical problems can create psychological distress [2, 9].

High stress levels can interfere with doctor ability to provide emotional support.

Patients who experience prolonged hospitalizations are at a particular risk for psychological problems [2, 3, 9].

Many patients reported that some physicians still do not consider psychosocial support as component of cancer treatment and may fail to recognize depression in cancer survivors [2, 3].

Therefore, poor communication between patient and her clinician has been identified as the first level that potentially contributes to healthcare providers' failure in the management of those illnesses. Evidences that support its effectiveness need additional research and more attention to psychosocial aspects needs in cancer from policymakers [2, 3, 9].

Many women diagnosed with cancer can be managed as a chronic disease.

New diagnosis results in patient not being able to listen well or to understand her medical situation.

When patient education has been found to be lower or among women who are young or unmarried, the physician's first task is to provide patient with specific information about her disease process and support her fear of having cancer [3].

Several physicians endorse a wide range of barriers with respect to the diagnosis and management of the disease: organizational or patient issues [2, 3].

The Pap test is the first step in cervical cancer finding. An abnormal Pap test cannot tell for certain if a cancer or a precancer is present. Therefore, the result of the Pap test will guide your gynaecologist to the next step: colposcopy, cone biopsy or endocervical curettage.

Colposcopic examination of cervix is done to look for areas of abnormal tissue if we have high-risk type of HPV, genital warts, biopsy of the abnormal areas, follow-up care after treatment, and so on.

Colposcopy is most often done when the result of a Pap test is abnormal. During the test, doctors can take a small sample of tissue called biopsy. Then, the sample will be observed under a microscope by a pathologist, who can confirm us if cancer is present or is likely to develop. Cone biopsy may be used as a treatment to cervical precancers or some very early cervical cancers.

Doctors should be familiar with two aspects of caring: expressive behaviours and instrumental activities. The first one provides emotional support to the patient and the second one involves medical treatment [3, 10].

In our care system, there is a comprehensive care plan based on the needs of the oncology patients.

Physician's technical skills are valued and respected by a proportion of patients. Healthcare professionals found that patients viewed competent clinical-surgical expertise as the most important component of doctor-patient interaction. When the patient trusted the doctor's competence, the result of this linkage can make the moment of diagnosis easier [3, 9].

Many patients are stunned by such news. Receiving such a message can produce questions as 'why me' and conclude that they are being punished by God for had acts of the past. Depending on the severity of the disease, a few patients may even contemplate death for themselves. Accepting the diagnosis and situation take time for most patients. It is important not to compare their disease with the others because that causes stress and pressure to themselves [2, 3, 9].

A considerable number of the women diagnosed with cancer are an intrinsically vulnerable population due to psychological factors. Women who showed less interest or lower intention to engage in cancer screening programs and women with lower educational qualifications or emotional barriers such as embarrassment could be associated with no improvement in the mental health status [2, 3, 9].

Some believed that women will only participate in screening programs if they are forced to do so.

What we can all agree on is that the absence of a set of practical clinical guidelines or incomplete recommendations on monitoring for psychosocial aspects of women with cancer put patients and healthcare providers at risk [2].

The factors who predict vulnerability to psychological symptoms or physical health should be viewed in the context of a cancer diagnostic as having high life consequences [3, 9].

Psychological factors have an important role in the relationship between perceptions about the consequences of symptoms and cancer diagnostic experience.

By applying patient health questionnaire or Zung Self-Rating Depression Scale, it was found that loss of libido, impaired sexual performance or menstrual disturbances would be predictive regarding the presence of depression in cancer patients [2, 3, 9].

Factors contributing to depression include patient's age, race/ethnicity and type and stage of cancer.

To diagnose depression, this requires somatic symptoms such as weight loss, appetite loss, fatigue or loss of energy, psychomotor agitation, insomnia or hypersomnia or cognitive symptoms as poor concentration, excessive or inappropriate guilt, suicidal thoughts or recurrent thoughts of death. Also, genital symptoms could be loss of libido, menstrual disturbances or impaired sexual performance [2, 3, 11].

Suicidal thoughts, psychotic symptoms or profound guilt can be associated with major depression [3].

The effect of the immune system on the course of the disease can be considered as a period of special need for body image disturbance, relationship difficulties, depression or anxiety [16, 18].

Patient's immediate question is likely to be: 'what does this mean for me?'

This is a difficult situation and they must learn to treasure every single moment. Instead of feeling awkward, they may go through this journey by encouraging themselves to open the conversation with doctor [9].

When you are dealing with something so difficult, the consequences can be unbearable [12].

4. Prognosis of psychosocial disorders in cancer patients

Patients with depression are more likely to have an adverse impact on disease prognosis [13].

The biological connections of the immune system have been suggested as the mechanism for disease prognosis [3, 14].

At the present time when medicine strives to be evidence based, the psychosocial disease course has always been an important factor in cancer prognosis and psychological morbidity [2, 3].

Stress hormones can influence the prognosis of somatic disorders such as cancer. Therefore, the psychosocial care of cancer patients remains a challenge [2, 3].

The survival rate after cancer screening programs has improved prognosis and the number of cancer survivors has increased in developing countries [3, 9].

Also, behavioural and social factors might affect cancer prognosis and the length of patient's life.

5. Treatment of psychosocial disturbances

Standards of care include preventive strategies and treatment recommendation plans for follow-up cancer patients [3, 4].

Despite the increased curability of cancer worldwide, the psychosocial need of cancer survivors is an emerging reality in developing countries [22, 23].

The cancer treatment, psychological treatment and counselling or social support all include challenges relevant to the patient [3, 9].

In principle, support to quickly facilitate return to work has become interesting for the healthcare system. On the other hand, no patients require being treated by a specialist who does not have expertise and are somehow not integrated into innovative diagnostics or procedures and do not have the ability to deal with any psychological discomfort caused by treatment [18].

Most patients need support, but they just do not know how or they do not have experience in this area. Unfortunately, there have not been much studies about social support including family members, spouses, children, friends or colleagues. Patients who have a lack of social support have a higher risk of depression [2, 9]

It seems that lifestyle modifications can contribute or confers a positive influence on women which has been diagnosed with cancer and need further examination and measurements [3].

Evidence suggests that physical exercise can induce compensatory behaviours that lead to possible impact in the mental status [14].

Psychosocial care departments of cancer services can be delivered depending on levels of depression or anxiety in disease stage or course of cancer in order to develop an effective treatment plan [2, 9].

It will be necessary to ensure that patients with pre-existing depressive disorders could be integrated into management programs in order to establish the most effective method of detecting serious symptoms in order to treat them or to improve the quality of life [2, 3].

The use of mental status examination and psychosocial screening for cancer patients can improve the detection of depressions.

The oncology staff needs to be able to deliver some level of psychological care that may be high at some point in order to improve the rates of detection of psychological symptoms in patients showing anxiety or depression and help them reduce the symptoms [3, 4, 15].

Providing psychological support and analgesic use is highly effective in reducing pain [13].

The use of nonthreatening terms to treat anxiety, fear or sense of loss of control has been shown to improve or provide psychological support for cancer patients [2].

Patient's expectations influence the response to treatment even before chemotherapy or radiotherapy is administered depending on local cultures and expectations. Those diagnosed with cancer should be led to understand that they can fight against cancer [3, 16].

Psychological factors have an impact on how disease affects patients and their tendency to catastrophize the situation [3].

Pre-existing psychosocial issues as unhealthy lifestyle, depressive illness or substance abuse have been shown to be very important in the progression of the disease after surgery [2, 3].

Also, inactivity or obesity is a serious impediment to improvement in social dysfunction [3, 14].

It has been noted that if cancer patients are allowed to develop behavioural dysfunction, then prescribing medication is not effective [2].

The behavioural dysfunction begins in response to the presence of the diagnostic of cancer [9].

Some patients have had good improvement of their mental disorders with graduated exposure therapy [3]. This is a process developed by psychologist Mary Cover Jones.

Treating the physical symptoms alone can exacerbate emotional issues in a substantial number of patients. Some patients are actually using antidepressant agents to treat anxiety or depression in non-malignant pain [2, 3].

Patients' social support network can greatly help reduce the risk of committing suicide and increased the quality of life for patients with psychological disorders [9, 17].

In addition, family members want to offer support, but they just do not know how to maintain healthy relationship [3].

Some people going through genital cancer treatment are embarrassed about the sexual or intimate changes [18].

In fact, most of the medical professionals avoid the issue of sexual changes because they do not have experience or enough time. Unfortunately, doctors avoid the functional aspects of patients' sexuality after cancer diagnosis or treatment because it is not a life or death problem for the cancer patients [19, 20].

Depression is associated with slow recovery and reduced rate of survival [3].

Treatment can include psychotherapy and pharmacotherapy. Psychotherapy involves counselling, cancer education or support groups, and pharmacotherapy includes the use of antidepressants [3, 6, 21].

6. Conclusion

In conclusion, the physician provides effective treatment, but fails to address and geared the psychosocial issues associated with the illness.

Healthcare professionals will need to improve their skills in the detection of psychological problems in the patients with cancer. They should know how to diagnose anxiety or depression in cancer patients [2, 9].

Physician can effectively help patients to live as normal as possible despite dysfunctional reactions, behaviours, thoughts, women depression or sociocultural aspects [9].

Furthermore, patient appears to be important for the effective treatment than to identify and assess psychosocial problems among women diagnosed with cancer [3].

It is necessary to define the condition more clearly by studying patients and their psychosocial problems. It is important to receive accurate information and understand all their options. There is no tradition of multidisciplinary team causing a lack of integrated data solutions on psychosocial problems which appears to be important for the management of the disease [2, 3, 9].

The success of the outcome and procedure is taking time to deduce the concern she has regarding her diagnosis, treatment and appropriate follow-up [3].

Standards of care include preventive strategies and treatment recommendation plans for follow-up cancer patients [2].

Despite the increased curability of cancer worldwide, the psychosocial need of cancer survivors is an emerging reality in developing countries [22, 23].

The more healthcare professionals seek to understand patient's experience of being diagnosed with cancer.

As oncology experts, they have to support patients and their families in navigating healthcare system [24].

Cancer patient's psychological symptoms need to be understood and integrate them within their cultural values, religious and spiritual elements [3].

Cancer care specialists as part of multidisciplinary teams assume the role of providing care of patients towards the end. Therefore, oncology professionals are essential for patients and their families [2, 9].

http://dx.doi.org/10.5772/intechopen.69160

Prevention and management of the psychosocial aspects of cancer, with respect to psychological symptoms from diagnosis through treatment and post-treatment care, have not been fully established [25].

Understanding the impact of psychological conditions can help physicians to advice patients by referring them to the appropriate multidisciplinary setting [2, 6].

Screening programs for distress may be useful among cancer patients [15, 16].

As a part of cancer treatment, psychological interventions should be included in the major cancer centres from all over the world. Researchers and clinicians have analysed the relationship between physician and oncology patient [2].

International conferences focusing on issues of psychosocial aspects of cancer visit prestigious centres and learn from their strategies, improving training for researchers and increasing international collaboration will lead to increased curability of cancer worldwide [26].

Doctors provide state-of-the-art treatment of cancer but fail to address psychosocial problems.

Author details

Eugen Ancuta[1], Dumitru Sofroni[2], Codrina Ancuta[3]*, Larisa Sofroni[4], Ion Mereuta[5], Lilian Gutu[2] and Emil Anton[3]

*Address all correspondence to: codrina_ancuta@yahoo.com

1 Research Department, "Elena Doamna" Obstetrics and Gynecology Clinical Hospital, Iasi, Romania

2 Gynecological-Oncological Department, Oncologic Institute of Moldova, Chisinau, Moldova

3 University of Medicine and Pharmacy "Grigore T.Popa", Clinical Rehabilitation Hospital, Iasi, Romania

4 Mammalogy Department, Oncologic Institute of Moldova, Chisinau, Moldova

5 Soft Tissue Tumors Department, Oncologic Institute of Moldova, Chisinau, Moldova

References

[1] Ganz PA, editor. Cancer Survivorship: Today and Tomorrow. New York, NY: Springer; 2007

[2] Chochinov HM, Breitbart W, editors. Handbook of Psychiatry in Palliative Medicine. 2nd ed. Oxford: Oxford University Press; 2000

[3] Lloyd Williams, M. Psychosocial Issues in Palliative Care. 2nd ed. Oxford: Oxford University Press; 2008

[4] Surbone A, Baider L, Weitzman TS, Brames MJ, Rittenberg CN, Johnson J. Psychosocial care for patients and their families is integral to supportive care in cancer: MASCC position statement. Supportive Care in Cancer. 2010;**18**:255-263

[5] Institute of Medicine. Cancer Care for the Whole Patient. Meeting Psychosocial Health Needs. Washington, DC: The National Academies Press; 2007

[6] Gregurek R, Bras M, Dordevik V, Ratkovic A-S, Brajkovic, L. Psychological problems of patients with cancer. Psychiatria Danubiana. 2010;**22**:227-230

[7] Mikkelsen T, Sondergaard J, Sokolowski I, Jensen A, Olesen F. Cancer survivors' rehabilitation needs in a primary health care context. Family Practice. 2009;**26**:221-230

[8] Edwards B, Clark V. The psychological impact of a cancer diagnosis on families: The influence of family functioning and patients' illness characteristics on depression and anxiety. Psychooncology. 2004;**13**(8):562-576. http://www.ncbi.nlm.nih.gov/pubmed/15295777?dopt=Abstract

[9] Watson M. Psychosocial issues in cancer. Current Science. 2001;**81**(5)

[10] Gamsa A. The role of psychological factors in chronic pain. II. A critical appraisal. Pain. 1994;**57**:5-30

[11] Stead ML, Brown JM, Fallowfield L, Selby P. Lack of communication between healthcare professionals and women with ovarian cancer about sexual issues. British Journal of Cancer. 2003;**88**:666671

[12] Brink TL. Psychology: A Student Friendly Approach. Unit 6: Learning; 2008. p. 101

[13] Taenzer P, et al. Influence of psychological factors on postoperative pain, mood and analgesic requirements. Pain. 1986;**24**(3):331-342

[14] Daniel de Araujo Brito Buttros, Eliana Aguiar Petri Nahas, Heloisa De Luca Vespoli, Gilberto Uemura, Bruno da Rosa de Almeida, Jorge Nahas-Neto. Risk of metabolic syndrome in postmenopausal breast cancer survivors. Menopause: The Journal of the North American Menopause Society. 2013;**20**(4):448-454

[15] Holland J, Weiss T. The new standards of quality cancer care: Integrating the psychosocial aspects in routine cancer from diagnosis through survivorship. Cancer Journal. 2008;**14**:425-428

[16] Ludwig H, Zojer N. Supportive care. Annals of Oncology. 2007;**18**(Suppl 1):i37-i44. http://www.ncbi.nlm.nih.gov/pubmed/17311821?dopt=Abstract

[17] Spijker AVT, Trijsburg RW, Duivenvoorden HJ. Psychosomatic Medicine. 1997;**59**:280-293

[18] Lemieux L, Kaiser S, Pereira J, Meadows L. Sexuality in palliative care: Patient perspectives. Palliative Medicine. 2004;**18**:630-637. http://www.ncbi.nim.nih.gov/pubmed/15540672?dopt=Abstract

[19] Stead ML, Brown JM, Fallowfield L, Selby P. Communication about sexual problems and sexual concerns in ovarian cancer: A qualitative study. Western Journal of Medicine. 2002;**176**(1):1819. http://www.ncbi.nlm.nih.gov/pubmed/11788531?dopt=Abstract

[20] Avis NE, Crawford S, Manuel J. Psychosocial problems among younger women with breast cancer. Psycho-Oncology. 2004;**13**:295-308

[21] Stolerman I. Encyclopedia of Psychopharmacology. Berlin and Heidelberg: Springer; 2010

[22] Kaplan M. Cancer survivorship: Meeting psychosocial needs. Clinical Journal of Oncology Nursing. 2008;**12**:989-992

[23] US Department of Health and Human Services. National Institutes of Health. The NCI Strategic Plan for Leading the Nation to Eliminate the Suffering and Death due to Cancer. 2007. http://strategicplan.nci.nih-gov/

[24] Cathcart F. Psychological distress in patients with advanced cancer. Clinical Medicine. 2006;**6**(2):148-150. Review. No abstract available http://www.ncbi.nim.nih.gov/pubmed/16688971?dopt=Abstract

[25] Hoff SR, Klepp O, Hofvind S. Asymptomatic breast cancer in non-participants of the national screening programme in Norway: A confounding factor in evaluation. Journal of Medical Screening. 2012;**19**:177-183

[26] Last B, Grootenhuis M, Eiser C. International comparison of contributions to psychosocial research on survivors of childhood cancer: Past and future considerations. Journal of Pediatric Psychology. 2005;**30**:99-113

Chapter 3

Colposcopy of the Vulva and Perineum

Marta García-Yuste González,
Ana Maria Muñoz Ledesma,
Mayte Navarro Monge and José Schneider Fontán

Additional information is available at the end of the chapter

http://dx.doi.org/10.5772/intechopen.68768

Abstract

Due to the normal histology of this area and the multifocal nature of vulvar intraepithelial disease, vulvoscopy is more difficult and less objective than the cervix examination. Basis of vulvar colposcopy as well as benign vulvar skin disorders that are usually found in a routine gynecology examination will be reviewed.

Keywords: colposcopy, vulvar, infections, trauma, Liquen esclerosus, HPV, VIN

1. Introduction

Colposcopy of the vulva—vulvoscopy—is an essential step in gynecology examination. However, it is not as systematic as colposcopic of the cervix examination due to the normal histology as this area and the multifocal nature of vulvar intraepithelial disease makes the examination more difficult and less objective than the cervix examination.

In this chapter, we will focus on the non-neoplastic disorders of vulvar skin disorders that we could usually find in a routine gynecology examination. Neoplastic vulvar disorders should need revised review in another chapter.

2. Tissue basis of colposcopy of the vulva

Presently, acetic acid is universally used as an adjunct to colposcopic examination [1]. As a tool for examination of the cervix and vagina, colposcopy is based on the variable absorption and reflection of white light off different tissue interfaces [2]. Mucosal tissue color depends on the amount of hemoglobin viewed at the tissue surface, which gives the tissue different degrees of redness. The degree of redness depends on the distance between the underlying vasculature and the surface, which indirectly implies the amount of cellular material (stroma and epithelium) between the vessels and surface.

How acetic acid works as a contrast agent is unclear. Although acetic acid can improve the surface light reflection by dissolving mucus, it can also modify cellular proteins, including cytokeratins and nuclear proteins. Lastly, it is believed (but not yet proved) that acetic acid dehydrates the cell, which removes most of the cytoplasm. After dehydration, the cell is left with organelles, cytoskeleton filaments, and nuclear proteins. The effects of acetic acid are transitory: when rehydration of the cell cytoplasm occurs, any protein alterations revert to their normal state [3].

Because acetic acid specifically modifies cell cytoplasm and nuclear proteins, the contrast created by its application to the cervical and vaginal mucosa depends on the number of surface epithelial cells, the amount of cytoplasm in these cells, and the amount of nuclear material in each cell. It would follow that more light would be absorbed and little light would be reflected if there were few surface cells with small nuclei and large amounts of cytoplasm. The effects of acetic acid on these cells would require frequent reapplications to maintain the dehydrated state. The opposite (more light reflection) would occur if the surface interface were to consist of numerous cells with large nuclei and small amounts of cytoplasm. The effects of acetic acid would last longer because these cells would have little cytoplasmic fluid to rehydrate.

Thickness of the skin affects the opacity, and it varies from different areas of the vulva. Skin of hair-bearing areas is thicker than the skin of other areas of the vulva. This is why histologically identical lesions may have different appearance when present on different parts of the vulva. Its prominent surface keratin layer does not provide a clear view of the underlying blood vessels. Pigmentation can also obscure blood vessels. Therefore, vascular patterns are less marked and less reliable than with colposcopy of the cervix. Vascular aberrations such as punctuations and mosaic patterns do not easily develop on vulvar skin. They are less common and can be practically seen only on the non-hearing areas. Thus, leucoplasia and acetowhite epithelium are the most frequent colposcopical manifestations of vulvar pathology.

3. Technique of vulvoscopy

3.1. Inspection

The clinical examination of the vulva should form part of the routine gynecological examination, thus enabling both the correct diagnosis and treatment of numerous alterations and the prevention and early diagnosis of vulvar intraepithelial neoplasia (VIN) and invasive neoplasias. A correct evaluation should include basic anamnestic data, a list of symptoms localized in the vulva region, and a careful inspection and palpation. The vulva should be examined in a systematic fashion to include the mons pubis and labia majora, the labia minora, clitoral prepuce, clitoris, perineum, and anal areas. Attention should be given in the examination of the vestibule to the hymeneal ring or remnants, to the gland openings (Bartholin's and Skene's), and to the urinary meatus.

The successive aim is to identify the main clinical aspects of the lesion which can be summarized as changes of color, presence of swellings on surface, and loss of substance. The critical evaluation of lesions should allow critical evaluation of lesions and also allow the gynecologist to formulate a diagnosis to propose to the pathologist. In this way, the collaboration between clinician and pathologist can contribute to progress in the diagnosis and treatment of vulvar diseases.

3.2. Application of acetic acid

It should be performed after applying 3–5% acetic acid to the vulva for several minutes using soaked gauze pads. Keratinization requires longer acetic acid application for effect and often renders typical colposcopic grading criteria useless. Colposcopy should begin by using the lowest magnification (6×) to quickly scan the vulva. Later, it can be proceeded to higher magnifications, as necessary, to examine smaller satellite lesions.

Acetic acid can cause acetowhitening of normal skin at the vestibule, normal variant of skin at the vestibule, and the normal variant of vestibular papillomatosis, which can limit its usefulness in practice. Any inflammatory condition of the vulva, including infection and trauma from intercourse, can cause acetowhitening (**Figure 1**).

3.3. Collins test

The test that uses a solution of toluidine blue to mark vulvar lesions is known as the Colling test. All foci of nuclear activity will keep the color and become stained. This may happen not only in neoplasias but also in the presence of ulcerations, lacetations, peparative changes, and

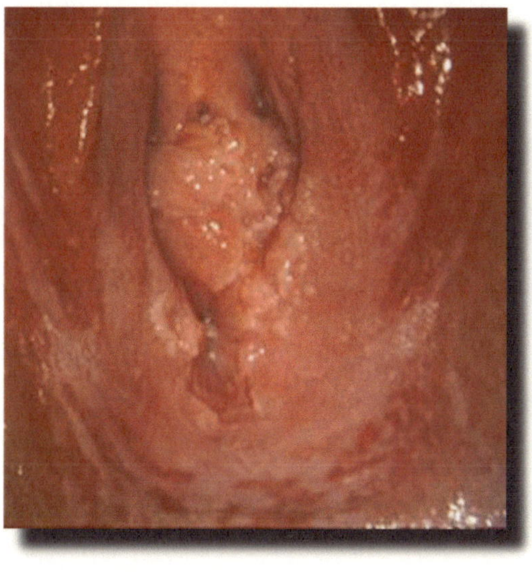

Figure 1. Normal acetowhitening of the vulvar skin.

parakeratosis. Historically, toluidine blue and Lugol's iodine solutions were used to stain the vulva and aid in identifying abnormal areas, but this practice has largely fallen out of favor because of high false-positive and false-negative rates [5].

3.4. Biopsy

Vulvoscopy can localize the lesion exactly. It usually cannot predict the histological nature of the lesion. Biopsy is indicated for visible lesions for which definitive diagnosis cannot be made on clinical grounds, possible malignancy, visible lesions with presumed clinical diagnosis that is not responding to usual therapy, lesions with atypical vascular patterns, or stable lesions that rapidly change in color, border, or size. Expert opinion is divided regarding the need for biopsy of all warty lesions, but biopsy should be performed in postmenopausal women with apparent genital warts and in women of all ages with suspected condyloma in whom topical therapies have failed.

Although information regarding the evaluation of women with immunocompromised conditions and human papilloma virus (HPV)-related disease is limited, human immunodeficiency virus (HIV)-seropositive patients and patients on immunosuppression after organ transplant may need biopsy of lesions when the level of suspicion is lower [6].

The area to be biopsied should be infiltrated with 1–2% lidocaine using a fine-gauge needle [7]. Epinephrine with the lidocaine can help with hemostasis but can make the injection burn.

After a test to ensure adequate anesthetic effect using fine-tipped forceps, a biopsy can be obtained using a cervical biopsy forceps, a keys punch 3–5 mm, or a small scalpel blade, depending on the size and nature of the lesion. Small biopsy sites can be treated with Monsel's solution or silver nitrate to achieve hemostasis. Only rarely absorbable sutures are needed. Location of biopsies should be indicated on a vulvar diagram or photograph, and multiple biopsies should be sent separately for pathologic evaluation (**Figures 2** and **3**).

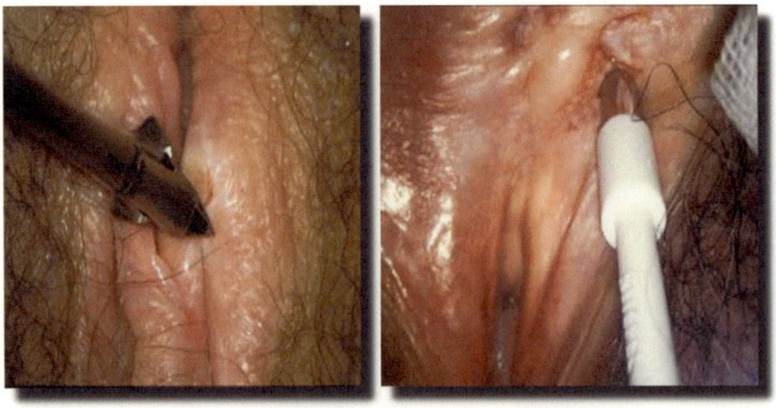

Figure 2. Vulvar biopsy with cervical forceps.

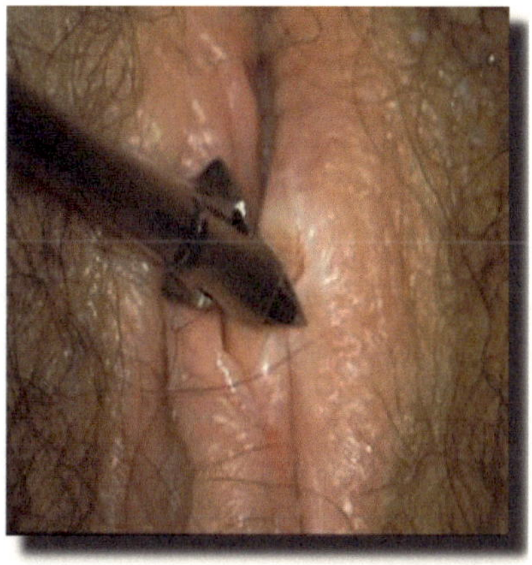

Figure 3. Vulvar biopsy with keys punch.

The simplest method is biopsy with cervical biopsy forceps, but an attempt should be made to get a specimen, at least 5 mm thick. Ulcerative lesions and very thick lesions should be completely excised to rule out focal invasion (excision biopsy).

4. Physiological hyperplasia (vestibular papillomatosis)

The etiology and clinical significance of vulvar vestibular papillomatosis (VVP) are still controversial; in the past, it was considered to be a result of human papilloma virus (HPV) infection, but actually, there are many studies that show only a rare relationship between VVP and HPV. Currently, VVP is considered as an anatomical variant of the vulva [8].

VVP was first recognized in 1981. A few years later, in 1991, the report by the International Society for the Study of Vulvar Diseases (ISSVD) described papillomatosis of the vulvar vestibule as the presence of multiple papillae that may cover the mucosal surface of the labia minora. Since then, VVP has been reported under a variety of names: vestibular papillae, hirsutoid papillomas of vulvae, vulvar squamous papillomatosis, micropapillomatosis labialis, and many others [8]. VVP has been seen with HPV infection, but a consistent association has not been proven. Therefore, most recent studies consider VVP as a normal variant in the vulvar vestibule architecture, not directly related to infection by HPV [9]. It is likely that this finding is a female counterpart of male pearly penile papules [10] (**Figure 4**).

Vestibular papillomatosis has been recorded in healthy young women in the range of 1–33%. The papillae of 1–2 mm diameter have the same color as the adjacent mucosa. The lesions are soft and are symmetrical or may be linear. They may cover labia minora and the introitus vaginae to a variable extent. They may resemble warts but are distinguished by the fact that the bases of individual papules remain separate unlike in warts where filiform projections tend to fuse at the base and lesions are not confined to the vestibule or the inner aspects of labia minora. In addition, application of 5% acetic acid causes whitening of the lesions in warts, whereas vestibular papillae remain unchanged.

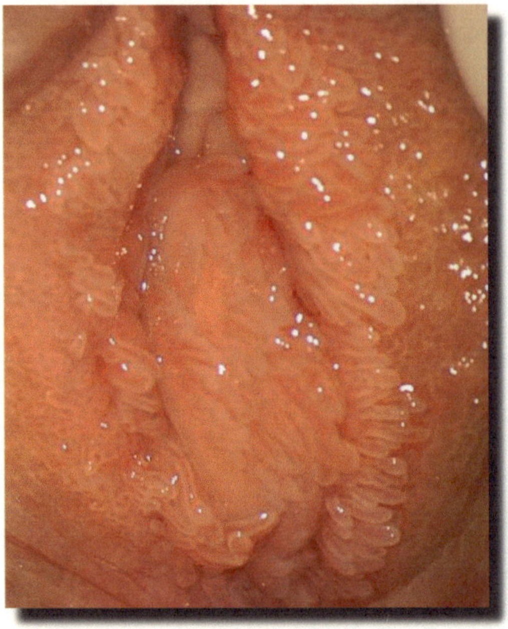

Figure 4. Vestibular papillomatosis.

5. Vulvar infections

Vulvar infections can be of variable location and multiple etiologies. Infections of the lower genital tract may be both specific and nonspecific, and affect the vulva more or less intensely. Some vulvar infections begin in the vulva and others in the vagina or nearby organs [11].

The external organs of the vulva include the labia majora and minora (folds of skin), the clitoris, and the vestibular glands. The basic symptoms of vulvitis are superficial red, swollen, and moisture-laden lesions on the skin of the vulva.

The characteristic symptoms are erythema, edema, pruritus, excoriation, and ulcers.

During vulvoscopy, color changes, topography, surface contour, and angioarchitecture of all parts of vulva should be noted. There are some vulvoscopic images characteristic of vulvar infections.

1. In skin, areas acetowhite and raised on skin, or areas with high yellow-white spots. If there is a predominance of reddish lesions, we may suspect infection by candida, dermatofitides, syphilis, erysipelas, or simply subcutaneous cellulitis.

2. In the mucosa, the infections produce an image of the mucosa acetoblanca and without being elevated.

3. We can visualize in the whole vulva injuries of the type of fissures, erosions, and ulcers of different characteristics.

http://dx.doi.org/10.5772/intechopen.68768

4. The presence of tumors of infectious component makes one think of infection in sweat glands, sebaceous glands of the vulva or even in follicles, or Bartholin's glands.

6. Bacterial infections

6.1. Folliculitis

Local infection of the hair follicle of vulvar hair by germs of the type *Staphylococcus aureus* or *Streptococcus*. This can happen because of shaving, waxing, or even friction.

It is described as an inflammation of the skin surrounding the follicle and erythema with elevation, small painful erythematous plaques, or palpation with punctate pustule. The treatment is usually local topical antibiotic, and in cases of increased dissemination systemic antibiotic treatment, penicillin derivatives such as clavulanic amoxicillin or minocycline and in topical treatment mupirocin.

6.2. Cellulitis

Infection of the subcutaneous cellular connective tissues was found below the skin in the vulvar area, and with easy extension to other areas through the subcutaneous tissue. The entrance of the bacteria can be from a wound or erosion or a frequent boil on the vulva.

It is described as an erythematous zone, warm and with a slight edema that affects the subcutaneous tissue.

The most frequent germs in cellulitis are *Staphylococcus* and *Streptococcus*. Group A strep (*Streptococcus*) bacteria are the most common cause. The bacteria enter your body when you get an injury such as a bruise, burn, surgical cut, or wound.

Their treatment must be with systemic antibiotic, clavulanic amoxicillin, or ampicillin (**Figure 5**).

6.3. Necrotizing fasciitis

It is a severe acute bacterial infection that spreads tissue through subcutaneous cells and fascia resulting in tissue necrosis. One-third of patients end up in septic shock with multiorgan failure. Treatment should be rapid with hemodynamic support, extensive surgical treatment, and systemic antibiotic therapy.

In the case of the vulvar region may be associated secondarily to surgical processes, such as partial vulvectomies, episiotomies of labor, or vulvar tears due to trauma.

6.4. Hidradenitis suppurativa

Hidradenitis suppurativa (HS) [12] is an uncommon skin condition that affects the vulva and other parts of the skin. The pimple-like bumps tend to develop in places where everyday pimples do not appear. Chronic inflammatory diseases of apocrine sebaceous glands are subsequently infected by bacteria such as Proteus, *Escherichia coli, Klebsiella, Pseudomonas, Streptococcus,* or Staphylococcus.

Initially, they are subcutaneous nodules that evolve occasionally to the formation of abscess due to bacterial superinfection and rupture. It can affect the skin of the vulvar region and fistulize later.

Early diagnosis and treatment can prevent HS from worsening. Early and long-term treatment may help control pain, promote wound healing, keep new lumps from forming, and prevent

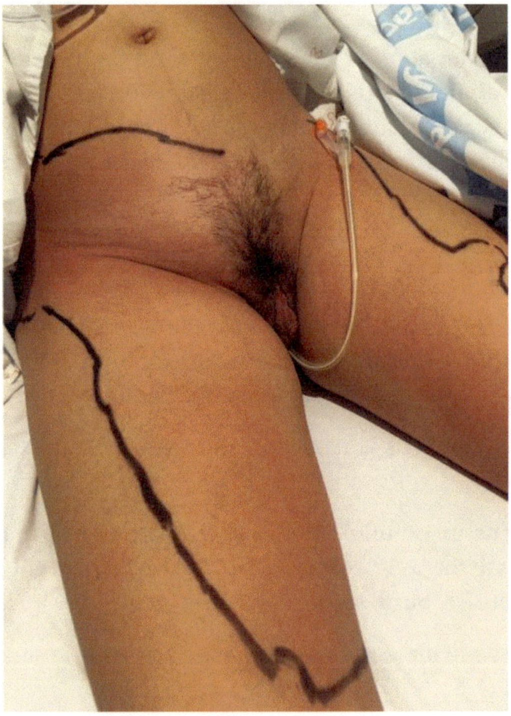

Figure 5. Vulvar cellulitis.

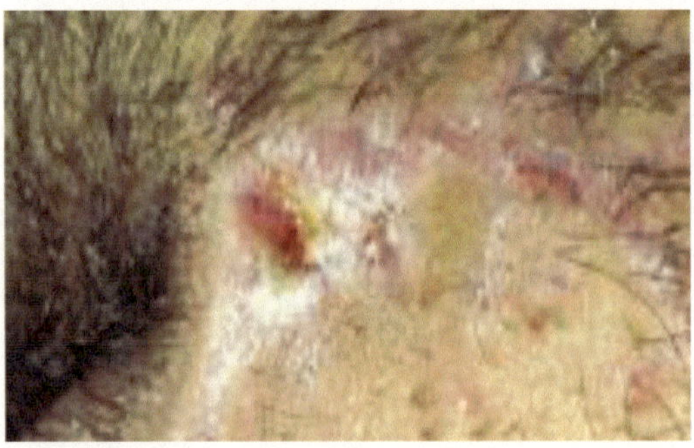

Figure 6. Pimple-like bumps in hidradenitis suppurativa.

complications. The treatment is surgical with drainage and associated antibiotic treatment, sometimes systemic, depending on the dissemination and severity of infection (**Figure 6**).

7. Bartholin's abscess

The Bartholin glands are located under the skin on either side of the opening of the vagina. It is an infectious process secondary to the obstruction of the duct of the Bartholin's gland that favors bacterial overinfection. Generally, the germs that produce the infection are mixed bacterial flora.

Clinically, it manifests as a tumor, with pain, blushing, and local heat.

Generally, in the acute process with surgical drainage with marsupialization of the gland or spontaneous drainage is sufficient associated with the use of oral antibiotics (cephalosporins, amoxicillin, and doxycycline).

7.1. Syphilis

It is a sexually transmitted infection caused by the mildly contagious *Treponema pallidum*.

The initial lesion is called primary syphilis. It is defined as the primary chancre being the inoculation site of the treponema, and after a macula appear initial papules that end in an indurated and painless ulcer, this ulcer is usually accompanied by an inguinal adenopathy. This lesion is called chancre and is defined as a firm, painless, and non-irritating skin ulcer, but there may be multiple sores. The initial lesion may appear on the vulva, vagina, or cervix. It can be kept up to 2–8 weeks and then cure spontaneously.

Secondary syphilis can manifest at 6 weeks or 6 months later by hematopoietic dissemination of the treponema. At this time, the characteristic lesions of the vulva are flat condylomas and erosive macular exanthema (**Figure 7**).

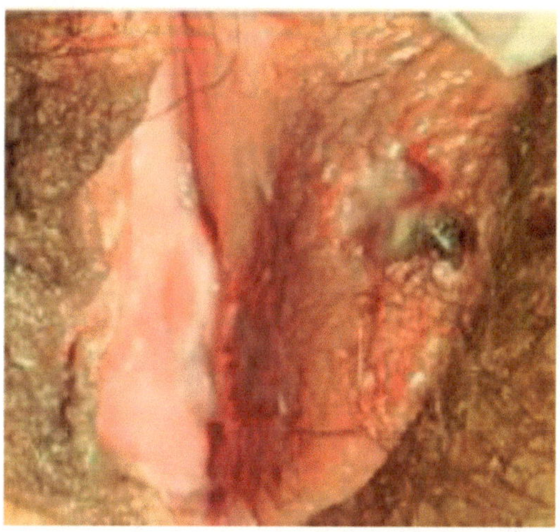

Figure 7. Syphilis lesions.

Tertiary syphilis occurs in cases that have not been treated. After a few years after the first infection, it is characterized because it has no characteristic vulvar lesions.

The diagnosis of primary and secondary syphilis can be performed with a microscopic examination in dark background, in which the spirochete can be visualized, and another diagnostic method is the serological tests, although these become positive in the late primary phase (VDRL and RPR or specific TPPA and FTA-ABS).

The treatment in any stage is with benzathine penicillin G injected into a muscle 2.4 million. In tertiary syphilis, we should use benzathine penicillin G intravenous.

7.2. Chancroid

Sexually transmitted disease is caused by *Haemophilus ducreyi. H. ducreyi* is a fastidious gram-negative coccobacillus bacteria frequent in the third world.

After a period of incubation of 5–7 days, lesions develop in the vulvar area, clitoris, or lips. With multiple painful papules surrounded by erythema, these lesions end up overinfecting and end up ulcerating. The chancre is soft superficial and surrounded inflammatory erythema with necrotic background. Not all patients are presented with this chancre, one-third presents multiple ulcerations that tend to unite and are accompanied by the presence of inflammatory and painful inguinal adenopathy.

The diagnosis is made by staining gram. *H. ducreyi* can be cultured on chocolate agar. The treatment is a single dose of azithromycin or ceftriaxone.

7.3. Lymphogranuloma venereum

Lymphogranuloma venereum is an uncommon sexually transmitted disease caused by *Chlamydia trachomatis*. The *lymphogranuloma venereum* is endemic in certain areas of Africa, Southeast Asia, India, the Caribbean, and South America. It is rare in industrialized countries.

It is characterized by a painless ulcerated lesion in the vulvar or vulva fork, which at 15 days is associated with multiple and acute regional lymphadenitis. In vulvar lesions, the most affected nodes are the obturators.

Diagnosis is by culture or arrest of antibodies.

The treatment is oral doxycycline or erythromycin.

8. Fungus infection

8.1. Candidiasis

It is the most frequent vulvar infection and is usually associated with vulvovaginitis. Produced by candida fungus, saprophytic fungus is usually found in the genital and intestinal tract.

http://dx.doi.org/10.5772/intechopen.68768

In our environment, the most frequent is *Candida albicans* and is estimated to produce 90% of vulvovaginal infections. Other less frequent but more resistant to treatment candida may be *Candida krusei, Candida glabrata,* or *Candida tropicalis.*

The clinic is variable and more in vulvar involvement, it may be asymptomatic, or produce pruritus attempt with erythema and vulvar edema. If accompanied by vaginitis, there will also be whitish leucorrhoea. In advanced cases, we can see papules and pustules with ulcerations and fissures.

Treatment is with local or systemic imidazoles. One should always think about discarding states of immunosuppression (**Figure 8**).

8.2. Dermatophytosis (Tinea infections)

Dermatophytosis (tinea) infections are fungal infections caused by dermatophytes—a group of fungi that invade and grow in dead keratin. Several species commonly invade human keratin, and these belong to the epidermophyton, microsporum, and trichophyton genera. They tend to grow outward on skin, producing a ring-like pattern, which coined the term "ringworm." The lesion is erythematous and itchy and extends through the folds and inner side of

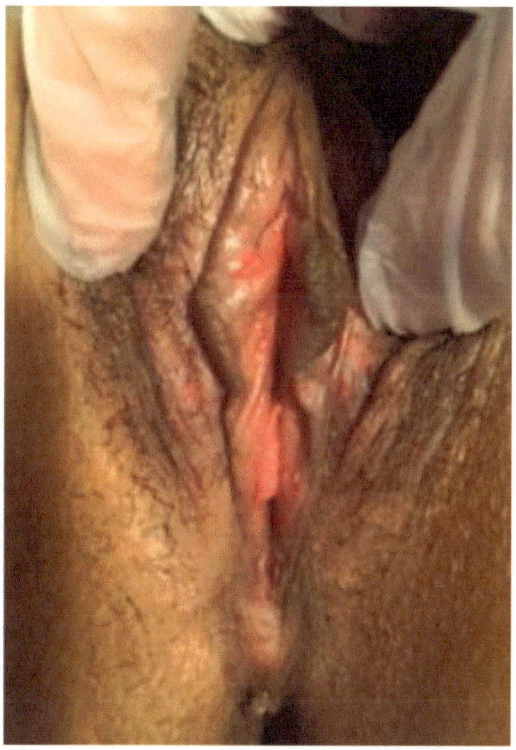

Figure 8. *Candida albicans* vulvovaginal infection.

thighs, also called margin eczema of Hebra. The treatment is with antifungals agents, either topically or systemically (through the blood).

9. Parasites infection

9.1. Scabies

It is an infection produced by the *Sarcoptes scabiei* or the itching mite that is a parasitic arthropod that penetrates the skin and causes scabies. Lesions are considered to be a skin hypersensitivity reaction to the parasite.

The lesions are lines or grooves that have a small papule at the end. It is very pruriginous and is accompanied by scratching injuries. The diagnosis is made by visualizing the parasite in lesions.

The treatment is with 5% permethrin.

9.2. Pediculosis pubis

Pediculosis pubis is a human ectoparasitosis caused by *Phthirus pubis,* this is generally consider of sexual transmission and variable percentages is associated with other diseases of this kind.

It is an infection caused by lice, *P. pubis,* in vulvar hair. Pediculosis is a very contagious sexually transmitted disease. The parasite can survive up to 24 hours outside the host.

The primary clinic is pruritus, and as a consequence, the visible lesions are scratch lesions.

Diagnosis is the visualization of the insect or nits.

Treatment also was with 1% permethrin.

10. Virus infections

10.1. Molluscum contagiosum

It is an infection produced by a Poxvirus. The transmission is by direct contact and it is frequent in children. In adults, it can be considered sexually transmitted by contact. The lesion is characterized as a pink papular elevation, that then becomes more blaquecina, is accompanied by an erythematous halo, the lesion is very pruriginous and is usually umbilicated.

They are multiple and of small sizes.

The treatment is with surgical or medical curettage.

10.2. Herpes virus

A total of 80% of vulvar and genital herpes virus lesions are produced by HSV-2 and estimated to be 15% HSV-1. Its prevalence has been increasing in recent years. Transmission may be by direct contact with ulcerated lesions or by relation to an asymptomatic person.

Vulvar lesions are vesicles in a different location with ulcers and erythema around them, characterized by being very painful. If it affects the urethra, it can lead to dysuria.

The diagnosis is clinical and confirmed by viral culture. Treatment is with Acyclovir, guanosine analog, or famciclovir or valaciclovir (**Figure 9**).

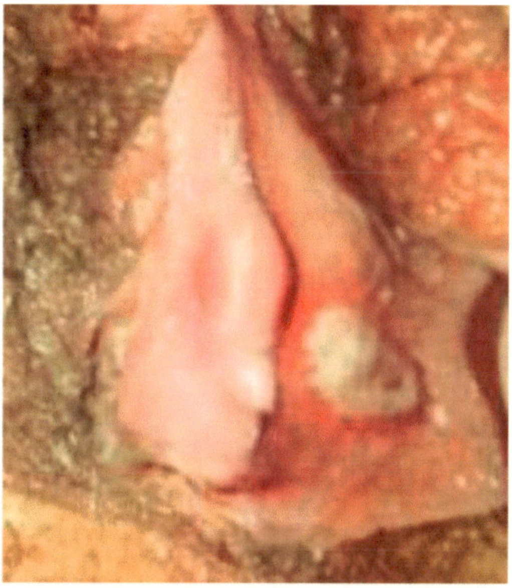

Figure 9. Vulvar herpes lesions are vesicles.

11. Human papilloma virus (HPV) infection

Papillomaviruses are a large and diverse group of viruses. It includes approximately 200 fully described types that have been detected in humans. Human papilloma viruses (HPV) are etiologic agents during various benign and malignant lesions of mucous membrane and skin epithelium. HPV is transmitted through contact with infected skin or mucosa. Very importantly, persistent HPV infection of certain types is a leading cause of carcinoma of uterine cervix, penis, vulva, vagina, anal canal, and fauces (including tongue base and tonsils). HPV infection prophylaxis is the best means to control HPV-conditioned diseases, and vaccination, as had been demonstrated, is the most effective method of its prophylaxis (**Table 1**).

A. Clinical: evident without magnification or acetic acid
1. Acuminate
2. Papular
3. Pamilomatosus
B. Subclinical: better assessed by magnification and acetic acid
1. Micropapillary
2. Flat
C. Non-clinical: evident by laboratory techniques

Table 1. Human papillomavirus (HPV) nomenclature.

HPV types are divided into low-risk and high-risk types based upon associated risk for cancer. The low-risk types HPV 6 and/or HPV 11 are detected in around 90% of anogenital warts, although coinfection with other low-risk or high-risk types of HPV is common.

Principle characteristics and clinical manifestations of papillomavirus infection are examined as follows:

11.1. Clinical HPV infection

HPV infection is the most common sexually transmitted disease in the world. At least 75% of sexually active adults in the USA have been infected with at least one genital HPV type at some time [13]. The estimated prevalence rate of HPV anogenital infection in the US adult population is 10–20% among unvaccinated individuals. HPV infection rates are trending downward in countries where HPV vaccination has been implemented.

Condylomata are relatively common. Reported prevalence rates based upon reviews of administrative databases or medical charts and prospective physician reports ranged from 0.13 to 0.56%, and reported prevalence rates based upon genital examinations ranged from 0.2 to 5.1%. Condylomata acuminate (CA) is the most common in young adults [15].

Sexual activity is the primary risk factor for anogenital human papillomavirus (HPV) infection. Once acquired, HPV infection can enter a latent phase without signs or symptoms.

However, only a small proportion of patients infected by this virus will express the disease. Nevertheless, this dermatitis remains one of the most prevalent of sexually transmitted diseases and poses problems in its management. These problems are centered on phenomena of viral latency, which do not permit one to guarantee the cure of the patient, and the absence of specific anti-viral treatment.

Immunosuppression is associated with the development of larger and more treatment-resistant condylomata, higher rates of recurrence, and malignant transformation of anogenital warts. As examples, condylomata in patients with human immunodeficiency virus (HIV) infection, receiving immunosuppressive therapy, or with diabetes [16] can be challenging to treat. Extensive anogenital warts have been reported in patients with human T-lymphotropic virus type I (HTLV-I) infection, and in association with the immune reconstitution inflammatory syndrome [14, 17].

Smoking has been associated with increased risk for condylomata. Risk for condylomata may increase as the number of cigarettes smoked per day and number of pack-years increase.

Male circumcision may reduce risk for HPV infection.

HPV may infect any part of the vulva, but initial changes most often appear on the areas traumatized during sexual intercourse. External anogenital warts are typically found on the vulva and groin. They often extend to the lower vagina, and sometimes the entire vagina is affected. Posteriorly infection might extend to the perineum, perianal skin, and/or suprapubic skin. During the examination, acetic acid is applied and the field is colposcopically examined.

11.1.1. Condyloma acuminata

Although human papillomavirus (HPV) 6 and HPV 11, low-risk HPV types, are responsible for most cases of CA, coinfection with high-risk HPV genotypes linked to anogenital and head and neck cancers is common.

In patients who develop CA, the usual incubation period is three weeks to eight months.

In most cases, clinicians familiar with the clinical manifestations of CA can diagnose CA based upon the physical examination. Findings that suggest CA are single or multiple soft, smooth, or papillated papules or plaques are limited to the anogenital area. The color varies: warts may be white, skin-colored, erythematous (pink or red), violaceous, brown, or hyperpigmented. Anogenital warts are usually soft to palpation and can range from 1 mm to more than several centimeters in diameter. The warts are typically asymptomatic but may be pruritic.

Patients may have simultaneous infection of the genital area and perianal skin. Therefore, all areas of predilection for CA (vulva, penis, perineum, perianal skin, mons pubis, and crural folds) should be examined. Of note, uncircumcised foreskin or hair can obscure warts, warranting careful examination.

The physical examination should also include an assessment for other clinical signs that may suggest coexisting sexually transmitted diseases, such as ulcerations, adenopathy, vesicles, or discharge.

If there is uncertainty about the diagnosis, a biopsy should be performed. A shave procedure to remove a suspected wart or sample a large suspected wart is usually sufficient.

In addition, a biopsy to confirm the diagnosis and rule out malignancy is beneficial for CA that appear refractory to treatment, especially in immunosuppressed patients. Other indications for biopsy include atypical features (e.g., induration, fixation to underlying structures, bleeding, atypical pigmentation, or ulceration).

Human papillomavirus (HPV) testing of warts is not routinely indicated for diagnosis. Testing does not confirm the diagnosis and does not influence management of CA [18].

Application of acetic acid has a low positive predictive value for diagnosing external anogenital warts. Therefore, use cannot be advocated for diagnosis [19]. False-positive results commonly occur, resulting from parakeratosis in other pathologic processes (e.g., psoriasis, candidiasis, healing epithelium, and lichen planus). The pain associated with acetic acid examination is another reason to avoid its use.

The evaluation of patients with CA should include a review of the need for testing for other sexually transmitted diseases and concomitant internal involvement.

Patients with external anogenital warts may have concomitant involvement of the urethra, vagina, cervix, or rectum.

Giant condyloma acuminatum is a rare tumor first described as Buschke-Löwenstein tumor. The disease begins as an apparently straightforward viral wart, but relentlessly enlarges destruction to surrounding tissue. It is a low-grade form of squamous cell carcinoma associated with HPV 6 and 11 that most commonly manifests on the glans penis, foreskin, and perianal regions. Giant condyloma acuminatum can manifest in large cauliflower shapes and can form fistulas and/or abscesses with local neoplastic invasion. Clinically, the tumor looks malignant, but in contrast to cancer, it does not metastasize. It tends to infiltrate underlying tissues and cause local destruction.

For women with limited vulvar disease who can comply with self-therapy at home, we suggest imiquimod over podophyllotoxin as initial medical treatment. For those who cannot comply with self-therapy or fail self-therapy, we suggest treatment with trichloroacetic acid (TCA) rather than cryotherapy.

Laser ablation is our preferred surgical approach as it is possible to reach into the vagina and the depth of treatment can be controlled (**Figure 10**).

11.2. Subclinical infections

Subclinical infections may be visualized through the colposcope after the application of 3–5% acetic acid. They are associated with intraepithelial disease (VIN) in 10–20% of cases. These lesions are distributed around the vaginal introitus, on the perineum and perianal areas. They can be asymptomatic, but in many women, they can cause pruritus and dyspareunia. Vulvar inspeccion will be normal skin, and colposcopically subclinical HPV infection cannot be distinguished from VIN, making biopsy necessary. Conservative treatment is recommended (**Figure 11** and **Table 2**).

11.2.1. Vulvar trauma

The etiological factors that can damage the genital tract are multiple and varied and range from births, coitus, foreign bodies, thermal stimuli, chemical, accidents, surgical acts and in another dimension, injuries or caused by sexual aggression.

The most severe forms that significantly compromise the anatomy or physiology of the genitals.

http://dx.doi.org/10.5772/intechopen.68768

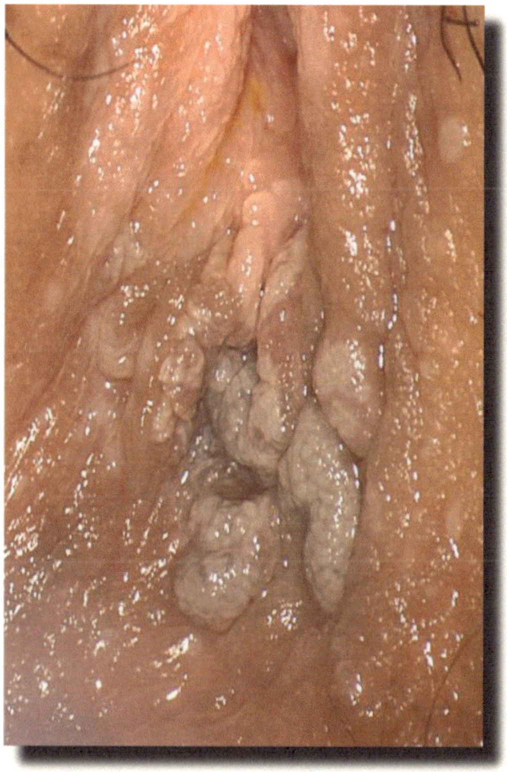

Figure 10. Vulvar condylomata.

The most frequent injuries are the direct ones and according to where they are located, we can speak of:

1. Hymen trauma: The hymen is a rudimentary membrane that is not very vascularized and can rupture with first relation or with the penetration of other objects such as tampons.

2. Vulvar tear: They can be secondary to sudden sexual intercourse or penetration of foreign bodies and usually have continuity with the vagina. Here, we could also describe the episiotomy or tear due to vaginal delivery.

3. Accident wounds are the most common vulvar trauma, as we have described before may be direct or indirect.

The direct ones are by falls, blows, or impalamientos with other objects. They are frequent in girls due to injuries with bicycles or blows when leaving the bath or pool.

The indirect ones we see them in great traffic accidents or collapses.

Treatment of injuries and injuries of the genital tract: It is designed to contain bleeding and plastic reconstruction of the injured organ if appropriate. The first will be done by ligating the

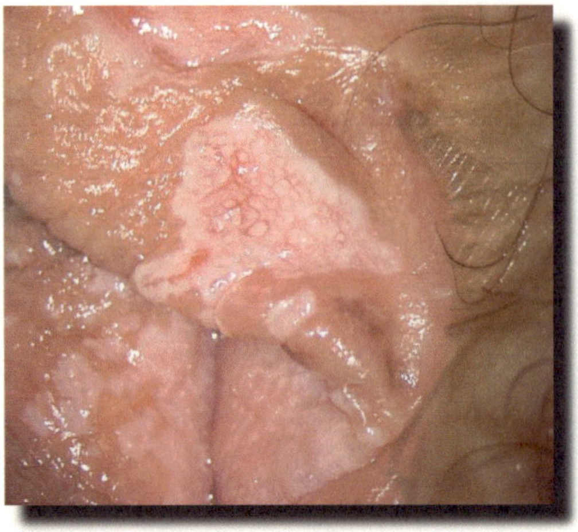

Figure 11. Acetowhite mosaic changes.

Feature	Low-grade lesion	High-grade lesions
Color	Snow white to bright white	Bright white to dull (oyster) gray
Lesion size and shape	Relatively large and geographic; raised and papillary	Relatively small; smooth and flat
Location	Throughout the ectocervix	In the upper transformation zone at or near the new squamocolumnar junction
Time interval to color change; number of reapplications	Slow to change; requires numerous reapplications to maintain color differential	Rapid change; requires few reapplications to maintain color differential
Border	Irregular; relatively indistinct	Straight, raised or rolled; prominent

Table 2. Acetowhite changes in low- and high-grade colposcopic lesions.

bleeding vessels that are identified or by hemostatic points. The wound will be sutured with loose stitches. There will then be a plugging in the area of the wound.

In the case of bruises, most cases require drainage to prevent the hematoma from dissecting the adjacent tissues by the tension they generate.

In all injuries, it must be ruled out that there has been no injury to internal organs either directly or indirectly.

The most common vulvar trauma is that produced by labor, vulvovaginal tear that may require subsequent suturing (**Figure 12**).

11.2.2. Liquen esclerosus (LS)

LS is a non-neoplastic chronic lymphocyte-mediated inflammatory dermatosis with distinctive dermal sclerosis and with a predilection for the anogenital skin in women. The true prevalence is not known.

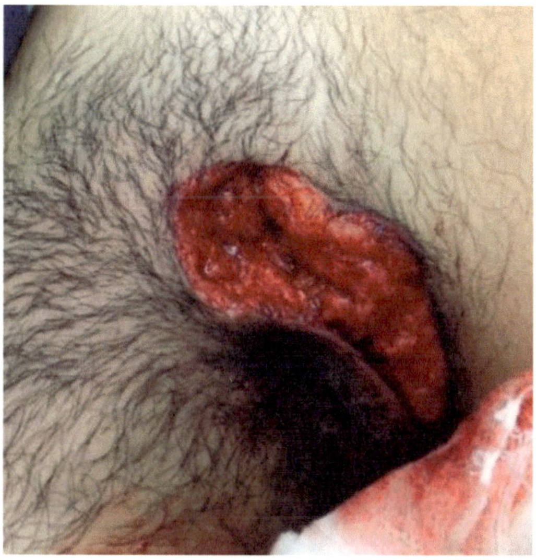

Figure 12. Vulvar trauma.

It usually occurs in the anogenital region (85–98% of cases), but can develop on any skin surface. Extragenital lesions are present in up to 15% of patients, although this may be an underes. Vulvar LS can occur at any age but tends to have two peaks of onset: prepubertal girls and perimenopausal or postmenopausal women [4]. It is one of the most common conditions treated in vulvar clinics. The true prevalence is not known; estimates range from 1 in 30 older adult women to 1 in 59 women in a general gynecology practice to 1 in 300 to 1000 patients referred to dermatologists timate.

Pruritus and soreness or irritation are the most common symptoms of vulvar LS.

Other women are asymptomatic; in these patients, LS is detected by careful inspection of the vulva for the characteristic thin, white, wrinkled skin, and changes in vulvar architecture. For example, there may be loss of portions or all of the labia minora, and the clitoris may become buried under the fused prepuce. Although uncommon, active disease may be asymptomatic.

Classic vulvar LS is expressed as white, atrophic papules that may coalesce into plaques, and follicular plugging may be observed in early lesions. LS can also be hemorrhagic, purpuric, hyperkeratotic, bullous, eroded, or ulcerated. The lesions most frequently affect the labia minora and/or labia majora, although the whitening may extend over the perineum and around the anus in a keyhole fashion. Extension onto the genitocrural folds or buttocks also may occur. Fissuring is frequently seen at the posterior fourchette, perianally, in the interlabial folds, or around the clitoris. The introitus may have a yellow, waxy appearance. Fordyce spots (small raised papules along the inner aspect of the labia minora, which represent normal sebaceous glands) disappear.

Scratching may result in excoriations and secondary mild lichenification (thickening of the epidermis with exaggeration of normal skin lines), often associated with edema of the labia minora and the prepuce.

The vulvar architecture remains intact early in the course of the disease. As the disease progresses, the distinction between the labia majora and minora is lost, and the clitoris becomes buried under the fused prepuce. Shrinkage of the introitus and perineum causes dyspareunia and more fissuring upon intercourse or insertion of a speculum. At the end stages of LS, the vulva is pallid and featureless due to midline fusion, which leaves only a posterior pinhole orifice.

The diagnosis of vulvar LS is based upon the presence of characteristic clinical manifestations, ideally with histologic confirmation.

Evidence-based guidelines from the European Academy of Dermatology and Venereology state that not all cases of adult-onset vulvar LS require a confirmatory biopsy. However, a biopsy may be helpful to confirm the diagnosis or to reevaluate the diagnosis if initial treatment fails or if malignancy is suspected.

An association between LS and squamous cell cancer of the vulva (SCCV) has long been recognized and thought to be the result of chronic inflammation and scarring. Much of the available evidence of the relationship between LS and SCCV is based on historical studies and retrospective case series. Risk has never been defined in terms of treated versus non-treated or unrecognized disease, or to the length of time the disease has been present. A 4.5% frequency of SCCV arising in LS has been estimated, with an average duration of antecedent LS of 10 years. This frequency is probably an overestimate. Earlier detection, the introduction of potent topical corticosteroids, the more liberal use of outpatient biopsy, excision of abnormally thickened skin resistant to medical treatment, and an increased appreciation of the nature and management of the condition hopefully will contribute to a reduction in the risk of vulvar cancer in women diagnosed with LS today. Those women who are not treated or have irregular treatment for their LS seem to be at a greater risk of developing cancer, although the figures are too small to be statistically significant.

Therefore, we recommend treatment of all women with vulvar LS, including those who are asymptomatic, to try to prevent progression of the disease. The goals of therapy should be resolution of the symptoms (pruritus and pain) and signs of disease, including hyperkeratosis, fissuring, and ecchymoses [20]. Atrophy and depigmentation may sometimes improve with therapy; however, scarring, if present, will remain. Clinical photography may assist in monitoring of the disease and can be helpful when showing patients were to apply topical therapy.

We recommend initial treatment of vulvar lichen sclerosus with a superpotent topical corticosteroid ointment. We typically administer clobetasol propionate 0.05% ointment or halobetasol propionate 0.05% ointment daily at night for 6–12 weeks, followed by maintenance therapy two to three times per week if symptoms improve. Thickened hypertrophic plaques may respond best to intralesional corticosteroid therapy.

In patients with persistent symptoms, we suggest a careful evaluation for causes of treatment failure (**Figure 13**).

11.2.3. Vulvar intraepithelial neoplasia (VIN)

Traditionally, squamous VIN was classified into three grades, analogous to the three-grade cervical intraepithelial neoplasia classification. In 2004, ISSVD replaced the previous three-grade

http://dx.doi.org/10.5772/intechopen.68768

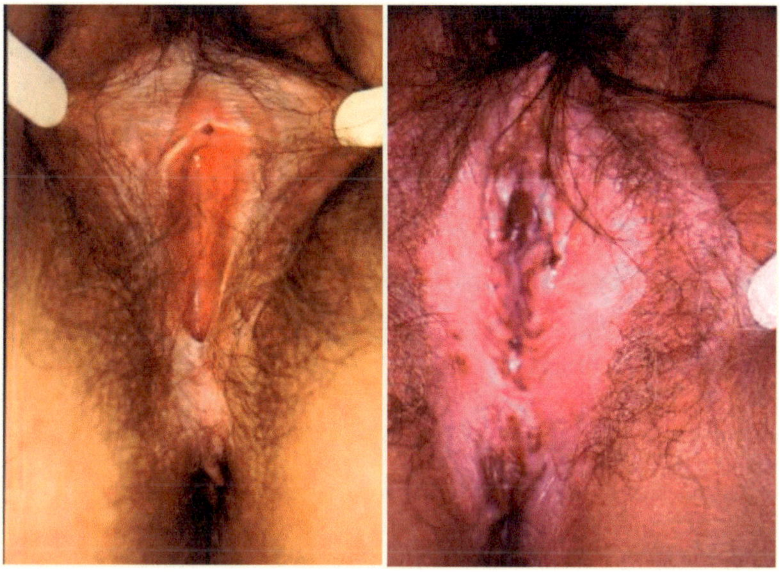

Figure 13. Vulvar lichen sclerosus.

classification system with a single-grade system, in which only high-grade disease is classified as VIN [21]. In that system, VIN is subdivided into

1. Usual type VIN (including warty, basaloid, and mixed VIN)

   Commonly, it is associated with carcinogenic genotypes of HPV and other HPV persistence risk factors, such as cigarette smoking and immunocompromised status.

2. Differentiated VIN: It is associated with lichen sclerosus and a squamous cell carcinoma of the vulva than usual type VIN. Furthermore, it has a higher recurrence rate [22] and decreased disease-specific survival from invasive squamous cell carcinoma [23].

Based on the 2015 ISSVD terminology of vulvar squamous intraepithelial lesions, usual type of VIN is now classified as vulvar HSIL, and differentiated VIN remains the same. Flat lesions associated with basal atypia and koilocytic changes (formerly termed VIN 1) are considered LSIL (condyloma or HPV effect) in the current 2015 ISSVD classification system.

11.2.3.1. Usual vulvar intraepithelial neoplasia (classic VIN, uVIN)

Basaloid/warty SCCs develop from classic or usual VIN (uVIN) which occurs more commonly, but not solely, in relatively young women between the ages of 40 and 50 years and is associated with high-risk HPV infection, most often HPV 16 and less commonly HPV 18 or HPV 33. In addition, uVIN is usually multifocal, multicentric, and therefore associated with other lower anogenital intraepithelial neoplasia including cervical, vaginal, and anal.

There has been an increase in the incidence of uVIN, and in some countries, the incidence has doubled in the past 10 years.

11.2.3.1.1. Gross findings

Low-grade uVIN presents usually as single or multiple pale-whitish areas, whereas high-grade uVIN presents as multifocal raised plaques or papules that tend to coalesce. A small percentage of the lesions (10%) may be hyperpigmented. There is a high frequency of mutlifocality in patients presenting with multiple lesions within the lower female anogenital tract [24].

Evidence exists that VIN III may progress to invasive vulvar carcinoma. However, the available literature suggests that the progression rate to invasive vulvar carcinoma is low (**Figure 14**).

11.2.3.2. Differentiated or simplex-type vulvar intraepithelial neoplasia

Although dVIN can occur in young patients, this type of VIN is usually found in postmenopausal women and tends to be unifocal and unicentric. Frequently, dVIN develops in women with chronic dermatological diseases such as squamous cell hyperplasia, lichen sclerosus (LS), and lichen simplex chronicus. In addition, mutation of the p53 gene seems to be an early event in the development of dVIN [25] with studies showing identical p53 mutations in LS and adjacent SCC.

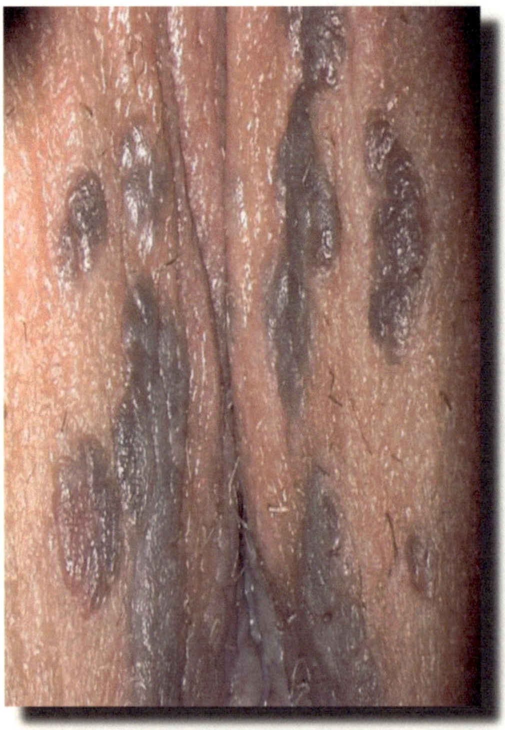

Figure 14. VIN: hyperpigmented multifocal raised plaques.

11.2.3.2.1. Gross findings

dVIN is found in patients with chronic skin conditions related to LS, squamous cell hyperplasia, and lichen simplex chronicus. However, clinical presentation is nonspecific with patients often being asymptomatic. They may present with focal discoloration, ill-defined white plaques as well as red hyperkeratotic lesions. Pruritus and pain are the most frequent symptoms.

dVIN has a higher risk of progression to invasive SCC than uVIN, and time of progression to SCC is significantly shorter in dVIN cases when compared with uVIN.

Author details

Marta García-Yuste González*, Ana Maria Muñoz Ledesma, Mayte Navarro Monge and José Schneider Fontán

*Address all correspondence to: martagyuste@hotmail.com

1 Department of Obstetrics and Gynecology, Hospital Universitario Río Hortega, Valladolid, Spain

2 Faculty of Medicine, Valladolid, Spain

References

[1] Powell JL. Biographic sketch: Powell's pearls: Hans Peter Hinselmann, MD (1884-1959). Obstetrical & Gynecological Survey. 2004;**59**:693-695

[2] Maddox P, Szarewski A, Dyson J, et al. Cytokeratin expression and acetowhite change in cervical epithelium. Journal of Clinical Pathology. 1994;**47**:15-17

[3] Burke L, Antonioli DA, Ducatman BS. Colposcopy: Text and Atlas. Norwalk, CT: Appleton and Lange; 1991

[4] Collins CG, Hansen LH, Theriot E. A clinical stain for use in selecting biopsy sites in patients with vulvar disease. Obstetrics and Gynecology. 1966;**28**(2):158-163

[5] Micheletti L, Bogliatto F, Lynch PJ. Vulvoscopy: Review of a diagnostic approach requiring clarification. The Journal of Reproductive Medicine. 2008;**53**(3):179-182

[6] American College of Obstetricians and Gynecologists' Committee on Gynecologic Practice.; American Society for Colposcopy and Cervical Pathology (ASCCP).

[7] Modesitt SC, Waters AB, Walton L, et al. Vulvar intraepithelial neoplasia. III. Occult cancer and the impact of margin status on recurrence. Obstetrics and Gynecology. 1998;**92**(6):262-266

[8] Rodríguez Prieto MA, Vega Gutiérrez J, Sánchez Sambucety P. Vestibullar papillae of the vulva. International Journal of Dermatology. 2004;**43**:143-144

[9] Beznos G, Coates V, Focchi J, Hatim AO. Biomolecular study of the correlation between papillomatosis of the vulvar. Vestibule in Adolescents and Human Papillomavirus. The Scientific World Journal. 2006;**6**:628-636

[10] Chan CC, Chiu HC. Images in clinical medicine. Vestibular papillomatosis. The New England Journal of Medicine. 2008:358-314

[11] Obstetrics and Gynecology 2011. Vol. 2. Usandizaga, De la Fuente

[12] Sánchez M, Torres JV. Hidrosadenitis supurativa vulvar,Vulvar suppurative hidrosadenitis. Progresos de Obstetricia y Ginecología. 2003;**46**:185-189. DOI: 10.1016/S0304-5013(03)75880-4

[13] Welch JM, Nayagam M, Parry G, Das R, Campbell M, Whatley J, et al. What is vestibular papillomatosis? A study of its prevalence, aetiology and natural history. British Journal of Obstetrics and Gynaecology. 1993;**100**:939-942

[14] Patel H, Wagner M, Singhal P, Kothari S. Systematic review of the incidence and prevalence of genital warts.. Infectious Diseases. 2013;**13**:39

[15] King EM, Gilson R, Beddows S, Soldan K, Panwar K, Young C, Prah P, Jit M, Edmunds WJ, Sonnenberg P. Human papillomavirus DNA in men who have sex with men: type-specific prevalence, risk factors and implications for vaccination strategies. British Journal of Cancer. 2015;**112**(9):1585-1593

[16] Hoy T, Singhal PK, Willey VJ, Insinga. Assessing incidence and economic burden of genital warts with data from a US commercially insured population. Current Medical Research and Opinion. 2009;**25**(10):2343-2351

[17] Weiss DA, Yang G, Myers JB, Breyer BN. Condyloma overgrowth caused by immune reconstitution inflammatory syndrome. Urology. 2009;**74**(5):1013-1014

[18] Workowski KA, Bolan GA, Centers for Disease Control and Prevention. Sexually transmitted diseases treatment guidelines, 2015. MMWR Recommendations and Reports. 2015;**64**(RR-03):1

[19] von Krogh G, Lacey CJ, Gross G, Barrasso R, Schneider A. European course on HPV associated pathology: Guidelines for primary care physicians for the diagnosis and management of anogenital warts. Sexually Transmitted Infections. 2000;**76**(3):162

[20] Neill SM, Lewis FM, Tatnall FM, Cox NH, British Association of Dermatologists. British Association of Dermatologists' guidelines for the management of lichen sclerosus 2011. British Journal of Dermatology. 2010;**163**(4):672

[21] Committee on Gynecologic Practice American Society for Colposcopy and Cervical Pathology. October 2016;**675**:

[22] Eva LJ, Ganesan R, Chan KK, Honest H, Malik S, Luesley DM. Vulval squamous cell carcinoma occurring on a background of differentiated vulval intraepithelial neoplasia is more likely to recur: A review of 154 cases. The Journal of Reproductive Medicine. 2008;**53**:397-401

[23] van de Nieuwenhof HP, van Kempen LC, de Hullu JA, Bekkers RL, Bulten J, Melchers WJ, et al. The etiologic role of HPV in vulvar squamous cell carcinoma fine tuned. Cancer Epidemiology Biomarkers & Prevention. 2009;**18**:2061-2067

[24] Yang B, Hart WR. Vulvar intraepithelial neoplasia of the simplex (differentiated) type: A clinicopathologic study including analysis of HPV and p53 expression. The American Journal of Surgical Pathology. 2000;**24**:429-441

[25] Pinto AP, Miron A, Yassin Y, et al. Differentiated vulvar intraepithelial neoplasia contains Tp53 mutations and is genetically linked to vulvar squamous cell carcinoma. Modern Pathology. 2010;**23**:404-412

Chapter 4

Colposcopic Assessment Among Women with Lower Genital Tract Pathology

Eugen Ancuta, Dumitru Sofroni, Codrina Ancuta,
Larisa Sofroni, Ion Mereuta and Lilian Gutu

Additional information is available at the end of the chapter

http://dx.doi.org/10.5772/intechopen.69176

Abstract

A broad spectrum of conditions classically requires a colposcopic assessment for either diagnostic or treatment means, including atypical changes in the cervix-vagina and vulva, abnormal Pap tests, cervicitis, polyps, cervical warts, genital warts, and bleeding. Although the procedure is commonly considered as criteria for the management of cervical cancer, the sensitivity of colposcopy is quite limited as its ability to discriminate among dysplasia and microinvasive carcinoma is difficult. Most professional societies and international health organizations have already released guidelines and recommendation for the management for woman with abnormal cervical pathology (e.g., cervical intraepithelial neoplasia and cervical cancer); only women with positive human papillomavirus (HPV) tests, low-grade squamous intraepithelial lesion (LSIL), or severe cytology have clear indication for referral to a colposcopic evaluation. While most guidelines recommend colposcopy for any abnormal cytology or any positive HPV test, others apply only for woman with two consecutive unsatisfactory Pap tests or for those with some abnormalities. In conclusion, cervical cancer risk remains high; thus, the potential benefit of colposcopy examination should be balanced against the risk.

Keywords: colposcopy, Pap test, cervical cancer, low-grade squamous intraepithelial lesion, high-grade squamous intraepithelial lesion

1. Introduction

When we have abnormal changes at the cervix-vagina and vulva, colposcopy may be used and the normal view is enlarged by the eye alone. Sometimes, PAP tests show abnormal changes in the cervix cells, thus colposcopy may be recommended to be done. Also, the procedure is performed to assess the results of a treatment or other disturbances: cervicitis, polyps, cervical warts, genital warts, and bleeding.

However, these techniques might have been expected to contribute toward managing women with abnormal cytology.

Also, the sensitivity of colposcopy is limited: the ability of colposcopy to discriminate among dysplasia and microinvasive carcinoma can be difficult. Cervical cancer prevention is a process using a combination between and biopsy, cytology, and human papillomavirus (HPV)-DNA testing.

The colposcopic appearances of vaginal squamous cancer may require biopsy for diagnosis because primary squamous cancer of the vagina is extremely rare. Colposcopists usually evaluate visual characteristics of the dysplastic lesions and cervical cancer. Once the diagnosis of the invasive cervical cancer has been established, delay in the treatment may carry a great risk of tumor progression. The procedure of colposcopy is used in the criteria for the management of cervical cancer and as a part of continuous professional self-development.

Most professional societies and international health organizations had created similar guidelines management for woman with abnormal cervical pathology including cervical intraepithelial neoplasia (CIN) or cervical cancer.

Women were referred to colposcopy only if they had positive HPV tests, low-grade squamous intraepithelial lesion (LSIL), or severe cytology.

Current guidelines recommend colposcopy for any abnormal cytology or any positive HPV test. Other guidelines apply only for woman with two consecutive unsatisfactory PAP tests or for those with some abnormalities.

In conclusion, cervical cancer risk remains high; thus, the potential benefit of colposcopy examination should be balanced against the risk.

2. Definition and why it is performed

Colposcopy is a procedure that allows physicians to examine the cervix, vagina, and vulva using a device called colposcope, which looks like a pair of binoculars mounted on a stand. When we have abnormal changes at the cervix-vagina and vulva, colposcopy may be used and the normal view is enlarged by the eye alone. The colposcope is used to determine the presence of abnormal areas. When the result of a smear is abnormal, the person performing the colposcopy (colposcopist) will be able to see problem areas more clearly. These changes are graded as mild, moderate, or severe and some are reported as "borderline". There is an adequate treatment for such changes depending on the nature of the condition. They could become cancerous if they were left untreated. Also, the procedure is performed to assess the results of a treatment or other disturbances: cervicitis, polyps, cervical warts, genital warts, bleeding, etc. However, these techniques might have been expected to contribute toward managing women with abnormal cytology [1, 2].

http://dx.doi.org/10.5772/intechopen.69176

It is now accepted that women who have abnormal Pap smear reports, CIN I, human papillomavirus, atypia, CIN II, CIN III, or even inflammation should be referred for colposcopy. There are many uncertainties and confusion about the significance of preclinical cervical carcinoma or changes in the cervix at a precancerous stage [1].

Also, abnormalities could become cancerous but this may take a number of years, and if they do it will cause alarm in women.

Inadequate smear results, postcoital bleeding, intermenstrual bleeding, and/or concerning appearance of the cervix are regarded as being reasons for women having referred for colposcopic examination. Also, it is useful for the evaluation of various vaginal or vulvar lesions [1].

3. What does the procedure involve

The colposcopic examination involves the visualization of the vascular pattern and epithelial opacity. The procedure means to look into the vagina and does not touch or go inside the body. Colposcopy can be expected to identify the area of the cervix called transformation zone. In addition, it is necessary to learn how the colposcopic examination can be made based on the natural history of cervical intraepithelial neoplasia understanding [1].

The colposcopist may wish to examine the cervix, vagina, or vulva and take a biopsy. This may need the injection of local anesthetic. Then, the biopsy is sent to the pathologist who will confirm the diagnosis of cervical intraepithelial neoplasia or cervical carcinoma. However, these precancerous changes will never progress further or can take many years in order to be reassured of having cervical cancer [1, 3].

It is possible for pregnant women to develop cervical cancer if they have previously had an abnormal Pap smear in the last 3–5 years. A colposcopy is a simple procedure that can be done safely during pregnancy; thus, colposcopy can be arranged. If the colposcopist observes any changes on the cervix surface, it is safe to take biopsies. The examination will usually be repeated until 6 months to check on the progress of the changes of the cervix. Because pregnancy can make the result of Pap smear difficult to interpret, cervical cancer screening is unnecessary during this period. Then, the procedure can be repeated during or/and 1–3 months after delivery in order to confirm the presence of precancerous conditions or to confirm the presence of cervical cancer [1, 4, 5].

4. Precancerous changes confirmed after colposcopy

Cervical intraepithelial neoplasia is graded as mild (CIN I), moderate (CIN II), or severe (CIN III).

Over the past decades, gynecologists and other health-care experts representing national and international health organizations identified strategies for the management of women with abnormal Pap smear and cervical intraepithelial neoplasia (CIN). These guidelines have greatly affected the optimal approach to hysterectomy in women with risks for cancer [2, 6, 7].

Cervical cancer risk is attributed to human papillomavirus (HPV) infection.

In agreement with other reports, an effective screening for preinvasive squamous lesions may be associated with adequate diagnostic measures, including colposcopic examination.

We can stop the growth of cancer development by using colposcopy to confirm whether it is cervical intraepithelial neoplasia or cancer [1, 2, 3, 8].

The abnormalities in the surface of the cervix are known as CIN. CIN indicates changes in the squamous cells of the surface layer of the cervix and rarely caused any symptoms.

Almost all Obstetrics and Gynecology Clinical Hospitals in Romania have the facilities for undergoing colposcopy.

The colposcopists may plan the treatment for most of the women who have abnormal areas at the surface of the cervix depending on the grade of CIN.

The cell changes that go deep into the cervix affecting one-third of the thickness of cervix indicates CIN I or mild changes. In order to find the grade of CIN, when two-thirds of the thickness of cervix is affected by abnormal cells it indicates CIN II or moderate to marked changes, and when the full thickness of cervix is affected it indicates CIN III or severe dysplasia to carcinoma in situ [1, 8–10].

Usually, most women who have an abnormal result at the screening test do not have cancer.

The Pap smear abnormalities are called squamous intraepithelial lesions (SILs). According to the National Guidelines, these changes are low-grade (LSIL), high-grade (HSIL), malignant atypical glandular cells of undetermined significance (AGUS), or atypical squamous cells (ASCUS) [1].

The high-risk types of HPV may be identified by HPV-DNA test. It can be done at any age for women who have an abnormal Pap test. The treatment depends on the degree of CIN and may include cryosurgery, laser therapy, loop electrosurgical excision procedure (LEEP), cone biopsy, or hysterectomy [3, 11, 12].

In most cases, the specialist may take a biopsy that may cause bleeding, discharge or pain, and cervical intraepithelial neoplasia. There are two different cervical cells in the cervix: glandular cells (endocervix) and squamous cells (ectocervix).

The aim of organized screening program is to reduce cervical cancer mortality by detecting changes in the cervix when they are still in precancerous stage and can be treated.

The percentage of cancers diagnosed during the program is an important factor, and leads to an increased willingness to participate in the screening program. However, some participants chose not to receive specific treatment regardless of a wide range of reasons. This suggests that the association between research and screening programs is the key issues for accurate measures of the benefits of cervical cancer screening [1, 3, 12, 13].

In distinguishing who will and who will not develop cervical cancer, it is the current clinical guidelines that matter.

5. Colposcopy as a diagnostic, screening tool, and gathering information

Cervical cancer remains one of the most common gynecological malignancies in developing countries.

The use of colposcopy is an effective screening tool for cervical cancer due to its high negative-predictive value. Some of the justifications against its utilization are the probability of producing unnecessary distress, bleeding more than you experience during your period if a biopsy is performed, chills, fever or severe pelvic pain, allergy to iodine and latex, infection, and false-negative results (the chance that women would develop CIN II or CIN III is low). Furthermore, there is a range of accepted thresholds including acute inflammation of cervix, acute pelvic inflammatory disease, and having your period.

Before colposcopic examination is performed, women must be fully informed about the possibility of the risks and other important information including no vaginal medication or tampon use, and no tub bathing or sex after the examination [1, 5].

Numerous symptoms that may concern you have been identified and include red bleeding, smelling discharge, fever, pelvic pain, chills, or spotting.

The colposcopist may confirm the presence of abnormal areas in the transformation zone as lesion size, lesion margin, acetowhite zone, and blood vessel pattern in order to select biopsy sites of the cervix [1, 11].

Among the limitations of colposcopy, we found that colposcopic sensitivity is known to correlate with the lesion size.

Recent data revealed that lesion size was associated with the degree of CIN and HPV genotype. Thus, smaller lesions are known to cause more false-negative cervical smears than larger lesions [1, 2, 6, 8].

Among several signs, the relationship between colposcopic characteristics and grades of CIN may make colposcopic assessment to have more benefits in the identification of preclinical lesions whose capacity for progression to cervical cancer has been demonstrated [1, 14, 15].

The European Federation for Colposcopy has developed a program of instruction for specialists and residents that should lead to a reduced number of cervical cancer cases.

We believe that the management of cervical abnormalities by cytology, colposcopy, and histological direct biopsy appraisal can help us to distinguish between low-grade lesions and malignancy that may affect the lower genital tract [1, 5, 16].

Both physicians and pathologists need to be aware of the existence of such cervical lesions to avoid unnecessary invasive treatments.

Developing countries have a high incidence rate compared to developed countries, so undetected pre-malignant lesions can lead to invasive cervical cancer [1, 15].

The colposcopic evaluation and careful examination of pathologic specimens showed that almost 100% of women with CIN contain HPV [1, 13, 17, 18].

It is now accepted that women with cervical abnormalities should be referred for colposcopy.

Clinical guidelines for health-care professionals are available for government organizations, professional societies, and researchers. These guidelines are designed to provide efficient monitoring and should help health-care professionals specifying actions to be taken to avoid or minimize the risk of cervical cancer. Most professional societies and international health organizations had created similar guidelines management for woman with abnormal cervical pathology including cervical intraepithelial neoplasia (CIN) or cervical cancer [1, 5, 12, 19].

It is possible that the number of women who have had a Pap smear in the previous 5 years is to be overestimated because patients who have had a hysterectomy were not excluded and reduce the frequency of colposcopic examination [1, 5, 11, 15].

In the case of screening program, guidelines will decrease the high frequency of the cervical cancer. Also, they showed us an improvement in the detection of intraepithelial lesions.

The ingenious conventional Pap smear or cervical cytology remained unchanged for over six decades. Most notable is that Bethesda terminology for cytology results had created the optimal screening guidelines in managing women with abnormal Pap smear results.

The Bethesda system has set the terminology and management for human papillomavirus-associated ano-genital lesions. The terminology should be relevant, uniform, and reproducible across laboratories in a wide variety of countries. This includes negative, atypical squamous cells of undetermined significance (ASC-US), atypical squamous cells that cannot exclude HSIL (ASC-H), low-grade intraepithelial lesions (LSIL), high-grade squamous intraepithelial lesions (HSIL), atypical glandular cells of undetermined significance (AGUS), and positive [1, 11, 20–22].

For women with LSIL, if the HPV test is positive or repeat cytology at 12 months is ASC-US, colposcopy is recommended.

For women with HSIL, if colposcopy is inadequate a diagnostic biopsy procedure is preferred.

For women with atypical glandular cells (AGC) and adenocarcinoma in situ (AIS), colposcopy is recommended in conjunction with endocervical and endometrial sampling [1, 11, 12, 23].

The Consensus Guidelines were updated by the American Society of Cytopathology. These are the result of a great effort to provide the current management algorithms for the world clinician's community [1, 13, 24].

The Bethesda system was the first to use the cervical cytology with patient history, clinical findings, and cervical biopsy to provide the best course of patient management and to reduce confusion among laboratories.

Most of the recent studies use the liquid-based technology in the detection of cervical cancer precursors. There are few clinical trials reporting a significant improvement in the detection of ASC-US, AGC-US, or adenocarcinoma [5, 11, 25].

According to the Cervical Cancer Screening Guidelines, the unsatisfactory cytology should be repeated, suggesting that colposcopic examination is necessary for those women with two consecutive unsatisfactory cytologies [1, 5, 11, 25].

More than 200 types of Human Papillomavirus (HPVs) have been identified based on their DNA sequence. In the case of cervical infection, HPV is transmitted by sexual contact. Also, HPV can be spread by anal or oral sex. Most of the high-risk HPV infections do not cause cancer but some of them may persist for many years leading to abnormalities that, if untreated, may develop cancer [1, 13, 17, 21].

According to the HPV type found in cervical carcinoma, the high-risk types, such as HPV 16 and HPV 18, are associated with HPV-caused cancers [1, 5, 11].

Some specialists are using anal Pap tests for men who are at a greater risk of anal cancer caused by high-risk HPV types. Several vaccines are currently approved by the Food and Drug Administration (FDA). Since 2006, Gardasil was approved for use in females. In the later years, the same vaccine was approved for men [11, 15, 26–28].

Is the risk of developing cancer following HPV infection in anal, penile, or oropharyngeal tissues many times higher than that following HPV infection in cervix? An appreciation of the HPV-mediated carcinogenesis of the high-risk HPV types and low-risk HPV types is still under investigation [1, 26, 28].

It is important to note that the majority of women with HPV infection of the genitalia including genital warts, precancerous changes of the cervix, and cancers can be treated.

HPV is a double-stranded circular DNA virus consisting of three regions: early gene region involved in viral replication and oncogenesis, late region which encodes the L1 and L2 proteins for the viral capsid, and upstream regulatory region (URR) which contains the greatest degree of variation in the viral genome.

HPV integration is associated with the highest degree of variation in the virus genome and with overexpression of the E6 and E7 oncoproteins. Instability of the host cell genome is the first step in the progression to cervical cancer [1, 28–30].

Several reports have indicated that the immune response plays a critical role in the progression from HPV infection to cancer.

The sensitivity and specificity of screening with speculoscopy combined with cytology were superior for large lesions compared to small lesions. Colposcopy is a diagnostic tool requiring time, costs, and special training; therefore, speculoscopy may be added for large or very large lesions in order to visualize the vagina and cervix [1, 5].

The colposcopic examination remained the recommended approach for identifying all abnormal lesions except for atypical squamous cells of undetermined significance(ASC-US).

Specific equipment for the colposcopic examination, the modern colposcope, is equipped with a built-in light source, binocular lenses, optical tubes, and the capability of course focusing and variable magnification through low, medium and high levels. Colposcopes may be equipped with variable magnification levels or single magnification so that colposcopists can have the best details. They have to take responsibility and avoid misguided interpretation of the reports [1].

The colposcopist and the pathologist should agree with the classification that will be given for cytologic or histologic interpretation.

The colposcopes are outfitted with an incandescent, xenon, tungsten, or halogen light, although colposcopy is sensitive for identifying the vascular pattern of the epithelium by using the green filter [1].

Recent technologies allow the examiner to identify the most severe lesions by a grading system that includes color, margin, and vessels. Also, the sensitivity of colposcopy is limited: the ability of colposcopy to discriminate among dysplasia and microinvasive carcinoma can be difficult. Cervical cancer prevention is a process using a combination between biopsy, cytology, and HPV-DNA testing [1, 9, 17, 25].

In a manner similar to laparoscopic procedure, video colposcopy will provide electronic transmission of data including demographic information and actual findings of lesions. However, colposcopists using video colposcopy should record the colposcopic findings including acetowhite epithelium, leukoplakia, mosaic, punctuation, and atypical vessels on the cervix, vulva, or vagina. The high-quality images can be scanned into a digital format for monitoring regression or progression of the lesions. All the biopsy instruments are specially constructed with a biopsy head and a handle shank [5, 15].

Performing the biopsy under colposcopic guidance allows the colposcopist to avoid misguided therapeutic decisions.

Tischler forceps may be used to obtain a larger punch biopsy with an adequate depth. Other types include Kevorkian, Burke, or Eppendorfer biopsy forceps [1, 3].

To achieve the acetowhite reaction of the epithelium, the application of dilute 2–5% acetic acid is required.

Lugol's solution would indicate that glycogen is present in the cells. When glycogen is absent, a keratinized area is present.

Monsel's solution may be used to stop the bleeding after the biopsies are obtained.

Recent reports have suggested that the main purpose of colposcopy is to assess the entire squamo-columnar junction between the columnar epithelium and the squamous epithelium of the cervix. The transformation zone was located on the exocervix in most cases of younger women and the endocervix as the age increased. This is the most common place on the cervix for abnormal cells developing [1, 18, 31].

There was significant correlation between the increasing number of live births and dysplastic lesions. This is because the transformation zone is directly exposed to external agents and the cells are more susceptible to infection. Pre-cancer changes may occur many years after first HPV exposure [2, 10, 20, 22].

High-risk HPV types include 16, 18, 31, 33, 34, 35, 39, 45, 51, 52, 56, 58, 59, 66, 68, and 70 types.

Low-risk HPV types include 6, 11, 42, 43, and 44 types.

The primary immune response to HPV is cell-mediated; therefore, immune suppression induced by transplantation or immunodeficiency disease may contribute to the persistence of HPV and the development of cervical cancer [1, 3, 5, 30].

Recent studies using quantitative type-specific polymerase chain reaction (PCR) indicate that human herpesvirus 6 (HHV 6), human herpesvirus 7 (HHV 7), and cytomegalovirus (CMV) are not cofactors in the development of cervical carcinoma. It is well known that the HPV replication begins with the entry of the virus into the basal layer and progresses to the surface of the epithelium. HPV in association with other factors promoting cell transformation may lead to a gradual progression to malignancy [1, 5, 15, 26, 28, 32].

Some researchers have suggested that CIN II and CIN III are the only true cervical cancer precursor.

In women with ASC-US, if HPV-DNA testing is negative for high-risk HPV types, cytology testing at 12 month is recommended [11, 12, 16].

AGUS is usually managed with colposcopy or cone biopsy.

In patients with low-grade squamous intraepithelial lesions (LGSIL), Pap test should be performed at 6 and 12 months. Furthermore, they should be directly referred back to colposcopy if cytology is unsatisfactory (ASC-US or greater). Also, if colposcopy is unsatisfactory, a Pap smear should be performed at 6 and 12 months with referral back to colposcopic examination [20, 22, 32–34].

6. Treatment after diagnosis of cancer

Microinvasive cancers are treated by excisional cone biopsy. Early invasive cervical cancers are treated with radical hysterectomy or radiotherapy. In addition, the patients can also benefit from concurrent chemotherapy [1, 3, 5, 11, 16].

Locally advanced cancers are treated with radiotherapy. Patients with biopsy confirmed CIN undergo standard practice for CIN [3, 15, 16, 24].

Several immunomodulatory agents, which have spectrum activity against DNA viruses, have been used as treatment for cervical lesions. Cytotoxic agents that arrest mitosis in metaphase also have the ability to treat genital warts [3, 14, 15, 24, 30].

7. Conclusion

The incidence of cervical cancer has declined in the last years due to screening programs that use Pap smear testing. The procedure of colposcopy is used in the criteria for the management of cervical cancer and as a part of continuous professional self-development.

Methods such as colposcopic examination and HPV-DNA testing have the ability to detect precursor lesions. Also, the improvements in colposcopy greatly facilitate the intervention on women at risk for cervical cancer. Cervical cancer risk remains high; thus, the potential benefit of colposcopy examination should be balanced against the risk. However, these techniques might have been expected to contribute toward managing women with abnormal cytology [1, 2, 5, 24, 30, 31, 35, 36].

In conclusion, the purpose of colposcopy is to assist the physician in clarifying abnormal findings and to exclude the presence of invasive cancer.

Author details

Eugen Ancuta[1], Dumitru Sofroni[2], Codrina Ancuta[3*], Larisa Sofroni[4], Ion Mereuta[5] and Lilian Gutu[2]

*Address all correspondence to: codrina_ancuta@yahoo.com

1 Research Department, "Elena Doamna" Obstetrics and Gynecology Clinical Hospital, Iasi, Romania

2 Gynecological – Oncological Department, Oncologic Institute of Moldova, Chisinau, Moldova

3 Clinical Rehabilitation Hospital, University of Medicine and Pharmacy "Grigore T. Popa", Iasi, Romania

4 Mammalogy Department, Oncologic Institute of Moldova, Chisinau, Moldova

5 Soft Tissue Tumors Department, Oncologic Institute of Moldova, Chisinau, Moldova

References

[1] Apgar BS, Brotzman GL, Spitzer M. Colposcopy Principles and Practice – An Integrated Textbook and Atkas. 2nd ed. Philadelphia; 2008. ISBN: 978-1-5160-3405-6

[2] Kierkegaard O, Byralsen C, Hansen KC, Frandsen KH, Frydenberg M. Association between colposcopic findings and histology in cervical lesions: The significance of the size of the lesion. Gynecologic Oncology. 1995;**57**:66-71

[3] Gage JC, Hanson VW, Abbey K, Dipery S, Gardner S, Kubota J, et al. Number of cervical biopsies and sensitivity of colposcopy. Obstetrics and Gynecology. 2006;**108**: 264-272

[4] Skoczynski M, Godzdzicka-Josefiak A, Kwasniewska A. Prevalence of human papillomavirus in spontaneously aborted products of conception. Acta Obstetricia et Gynecologica Scandinavica. 2011;**90**:1402-1405

[5] Wright TC Jr, Cox JT, Massad LS, et al. 2001 consensus guidelines for the management of women with cervical cytological abnormalities. The Journal of the American Medical Association. 2002;**287**:2120-2129.19

[6] Jarmulowicz MR, Jenkins D, Barton SE, Goodall AL, Hollingworth A, Singer A. Cytological status and lesion size: A further dimension in cervical intraepithelial neoplasia. British Journal of Obstetrics and Gynaecology. 1989;**96**:1061-1066

[7] Walker JL, Wang SS, Schiffman M, et al. Predicting absolute risk of CIN3 during post-colposcopic follow-up: Results from the ASCUS-LSIL. Triage Study (ALTS). American Journal of Obstetrics and Gynaecology. 2006;**195**:341-348

[8] Shafi MI, Finn CB, Luesley DM, Jordan JA, Dunn J. Lesion size and histology of atypical cervical transformation zone. British Journal of Obstetrics and Gynaecology. 1991;**98**:490-492

[9] Paraskevaidis E, Arbyn M, Sotiriadis A, Diakomanolis E, Martin-Hirsch P, Koliopoulos G, et al. The role of HPV DNA testing in the follow-up period after treatment for CIN: A systematic review of the literature. Cancer Treatment Reviews. 2004;**30**:205-211

[10] Schleht NF, Platt RW, Duarte-Franko E, Costa MC, Sobrinho JP, Prado JK, et al. Human papillomavirus infection and time to progression and regression of cervical intraepithelial neoplasia. Journal of the National Cancer Institute. 2003;**95**:1336-1343

[11] Wright TC Jr, Massad LS, Dunton CJ, Spitzer M, Wilkinson EJ, Solomon D. 2006 consensus guidelines for the management of women with abnormal cervical screening tests. Journal of Lower Genital Tract Disease. 2007;**11**(4):201-222

[12] Davey DD, Cox JT, Austin RM, Birdsong G, Colgan TJ, Howel LP, et al. Cervical cytology specimen adequacy: Updated patient management guidelines. Journal of Lower Genital Tract Disease. 2008;**12**:71-81

[13] Ronnet BM, Manos MM, Ransley JE, Fetterman BJ, Kinney WK, Hurley LB, Ngai JS, Kurman RJ, Sherman ME. Atypical glandular cells of undetermined significance (AGUS): Cytopathologic features, histopathologic results, and human papillomavirus DNA detection. Human Pathology. 1999;**30**:816-825

[14] Plummer M, Schiffman M, Castle P, et al. A 2-year prospective study of human papillomavirus persistence among women with a cytological diagnosis of atypical squamous cells of undetermined significance or low-grade squamous intraepithelial lesion. Journal of Infectious Disease. 2007;**195**(11):1582-1589

[15] Moyer VA, LeFevre ML, Siu AL, Bibbins-Domingo K, Curry SJ, Flores G, US Preventive Services Task Force et al. Screening for cervical cancer: U.S. Preventive Services Task Force recommendation statement. Annals of Internal Medicine. 2012;**156**:880-891

[16] Stoler MH, Schiffman M. Interobserver reproducibility of cervical cytologic and histologic interpretations: Realistic estimates from the ASCUS-LSIL Triage Study. The Journal of the American Medical Association. 2001;**285**:1500-1505

[17] Manos MM, Kinney WK, Hurley LB, Sherman ME, Shieh-Ngai J, Sherman RJ, Ramsey JE, Fetterman BJ, Hartinger JS, Mc Intosh KM, Pawlik GF, Hiatt RA. Identifying women with cervical neoplasia: Using human papillomavirus DNA testing for equivocal Papanicolaou results. The Journal of the American Medical Association. 1999;**281**:1605-1610

[18] Walboomers JMM, Jacobs MV, Manos MM, Bosch FX, Kummer JA, Shah KV, Snijders PJF, Peto J, Meijer CJLM, Munoz N. Human papillomavirus is a necessary cause of invasive cervical cancer worldwide. Journal of. Pathology. **189**:12-19

[19] Baum M, Rader J, Gibb R, McAlister R, Powell M, Mutch D, et al. Colposcopic accuracy of obstetrics and gynecology residents. Gynecologic Oncology. 2006;**103**:966-970

[20] Ronco G, Cuzick J, Segnan N, Brezzi S, Carozzi F, Folicaldi S, et al. HPV triage for low grade (L-SIL) cytology is appropriate for women over 35 in mass cervical cancer screening using liquid based cytology. European Journal of Cancer. 2007;**43**:476-480

[21] Maucort-Boulch D, Plummer M, Castle PE, Demuth F, Safaeian M, Wheeler CM, et al. Predictors of human papillomavirus persistence among women with equivocal or mildly abnormal cytology. International Journal of Cancer. 2010;**126**:684-491

[22] Datta SD, Koutsky LA, Ratelle S, Unger ER, Shlay J, McClain T, et al. Human papillomavirus infection and cervical cytology in women screened for cervical cancer in the United States, 2003-2005. Annals of Internal Medicine. 2008;**148**:493-450

[23] Shlay JC, Dunn T, Byers T, et al. Prediction of cervical intraepithelial neoplasia grade 2-3 using risk assessment and human papillomavirus testing in women with atypia on Papanicolaou smears. Obstetrics and Gynecology. 2000;**96**:410-416

[24] Renshaw AA, Mody DR, Styer P, et al. Papanicolaou tests with mixed high-grade and low-grade squamous intraepithelial lesion features: Distinct performance in the College of American Pathologists Interlaboratory Comparison Program in Cervicovaginal Cytopathology. Archives of Pathology and Laboratory Medicine. 2006;**130**:456-459

[25] Elumir-Tanner L, Doraty M. Management of Papanicolaou test results that lack endocervical cells. The Canadian Medical Association Journal. 2011;**183**:563-568

[26] Harper DM, Franco EL, Wheeler C, et al. Efficacy of a bivalent L1 virus-like particle vaccine in prevention of infection with human papillomavirus 16 and 18 in young women: A randomized controlled trial. Lancet. 2004;**364**:1757-1765

[27] Garland S, Avila MH, Wheeler CM, et al. Quadrivalent vaccine against human papilloma virus to prevent anogenital diseases. The New England Journal of Medicine. 2007;**356**:192801943

[28] Moscicki AB, Cox JT. Practice improvement in cervical screening and management (PICSM): Symposium on management of cervical abnormalities in adolescents and young women. Journal of Lower Genital Tract Disease. 2010;**14**:73-80

[29] Srodon M, Parry Dilworth H, Ronnett BM. Atypical squamous cells, cannot exclude high-grade squamous intraepithelial lesion: Diagnostic performance, human papillomavirus testing, and follow-up results. Cancer (Cancer Cytopathology). 2006;**108**:32-38

[30] Gage JC, Schiffman M, Solomon D, Wheeler CM, Castle PE. Comparison of measurements of human papillomavirus persistence for postcolposcopic surveillance for cervical precancerous lesions. Cancer Epidemiology Biomarkers and Prevention. 2010;**19**:1668-1674

[31] Dobec M, Bannwart F, Kaeppeli F, Cassinotti P. Automation of the linear array HPV genotyping test and its application for routine typing of human papillomaviruses in cervical specimens of women without cytological abnormalities in Switzerland. Journal of Clinical Virology. 2009;**45**:23-27

[32] Chan PK, Chan WW, Li DP, Chan JL, Cheung AF. Association of human beta-herpesviruses with the development of cervical cancer: Bystanders. 2001

[33] Solomon D, Davey D, Kurman R, et al. The 2001 Bethesda System: Terminology for reporting results of cervical cytology. The Journal of the American Medical Association. 2002;**287**:2114-2119

[34] Liman AK, Giampoli EJ, Bonfiglio TA. Should women with atypical squamous cells, cannot exclude high grade squamous intraepithelial lesion, receive reflex human papillomavirus-DNA testing? Cancer. 2005;**105**:457-460

[35] Rodriguez D, Christopoulos P, Martins N, Pargmae P, Werner H. Working conditions survey and trainees situation: New approach to auditing the situation of European trainees in obstetrics and gynaecology ten years later. European Journal of Obstetrics, Gynecology and Reproductive Biology. 2009;**147**:130-134

[36] Kinney WK, Manos MM, Hurley LB, et al. Where's the high grade cervical neoplasia? The importance of minimally abnormal Papanicolaou diagnoses. Obstetrics and Gynecology. 1998;**91**:973-976

Chapter 5

Utility of Colposcopy: Comparison of Colposcopic Abnormality with Histology and Cytology, with Colposcopic Findings Focusing on the Lesion in Cervical Canal

Hiroyuki Kuramoto and Toshiko Jobo

Additional information is available at the end of the chapter

http://dx.doi.org/10.5772/intechopen.68358

Abstract

This chapter discusses four significant items: (1) incidences of abnormal colposcopy in healthy women, (2) comparison of its abnormality with histology and (3) cytology, and (4) colposcopic findings focused on the lesions in cervical canal to prevent misdiagnosis.

1. The incidence of atypical colposcopic findings (ACF) was 3.6%, whereas that of abnormal cytology (≧ASC-US: Atypical Squamous Cells with Undetermined Significance) was 1.1%. The former is more frequent than the latter.
2. The incidence of unsatisfactory colposcopic findings (UCF) was high (24.2%). Pap smear is more useful in primary screening, if performed satisfactorily.
3. Colposcopy detects squamous intraepithelial lesions (SILs) constantly regardless of the severity of lesions. In cytology, it is easier to miss the lower lesions.
4. The incidence of benign reparatory lesion was 61.4% among women (n = 1317) who had either abnormal cytology or colposcopy and was 74.6% if cytology is negative. We should realize that colposcopic abnormality does not always show neoplastic lesions.
5. Main colposcopic abnormalities were the triad of mosaic, punctation, and aceto-white epithelium, which appeared admixed in the majority of cases with tendency of lesion severity. However, colposcopic abnormal findings in benign lesions are also the triad, although the admixed ones are few.
6. The abnormal areas were wider in order of severity of SILs.

Keywords: colposcopy, cytology, Pap smear, colposcopy-guided biopsy, cervical cancer, screening for uterine cervix

---

1. Introduction

Cytological smear taken from the cervix (Pap smear) has been a useful tool for the primary screening of the cervix. However, the sensitivity of cytology is not always high to detect milder squamous intraepithelial lesions (SILs, i.e., mild and moderate dysplasia) [1, 2]. It is clarified that cancer of the cervix originates from human papillomavirus (HPV) infection [3]. Accordingly, the introduction of HPV testing has been suggested as the useful strategy for screening for this cancer [4, 5]. Therefore, the standard screening method for this type of cancer shall be to use Pap smear with a simultaneous or ancillary HPV test as the primary screening method, and colposcopy shall be reserved for the detailed examination.

Medical institutions in Japan including ours, and Central and Eastern Europe, including Hungary, have had a long history of the cancer detection program for the uterine cervix, using simultaneous cervical cytology and colposcopy [6, 7]. Therefore, data from the program with simultaneous screening with cytology and colposcopy may be a good model for comparing the two methods.

In this chapter, we report the characteristics of colposcopy and cytology based on the colposcopy-guided biopsy and discuss three significant items: (1) incidences of unsatisfactory and abnormal colposcopic findings in healthy women, (2) comparison of colposcopic abnormality with histology, and (3) cytology. In addition, (4) we also show colposcopic photos focusing on the lesions localized in the cervical canal, which is easily missed to be detected.

2. Incidences of colposcopic utility and abnormality in healthy women

2.1. Incidences of unsatisfactory colposcopic findings

Cancer of the cervix originates at the squamocolumnar junction (SCJ), where layers of squamous cells and columnar cells come into contact with each other. Therefore, the SCJ should be visualized on colposcopy, and cellular samples for Pap smear should be correctly obtained from the SCJ area when screening is performed. The result of colposcopy is categorized as unsatisfactory colposcopic findings (UCF) if the SCJ is not visible. The incidence of UCF was 24.2% in total (n = 1967, **Figure 1**) and 20.3% in women (n = 1313) with a history of vaginal delivery, whereas in women (n = 97) with a history of Cesarean Section (CS) and those (n = 557) who had no history of delivery, these were 53.6% and 28.2%, respectively [7].

In other words, at least one out of every four women shows unsatisfactory findings on colposcopy. The incidence of UCF was high in the present series, although it has been generally considered to a range from 10 to 15%. This may be due to the increasing older age group in the

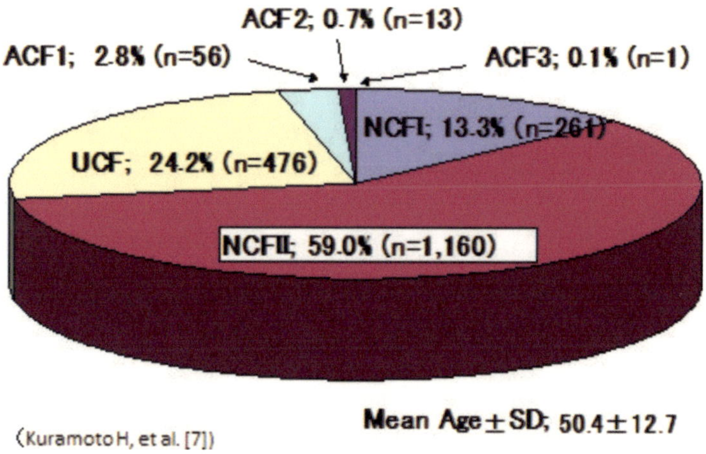

Figure 1. Distribution of colposcopic findings in healthy women (n = 1967) [7].

Japanese population. The mean age of the present series was 50.4 ± 12.7. The results suggest that colposcopy is not suitable for primary screening for cervical cancer. In contrast, there were no unsatisfactory Pap smear results in this series.

2.2. Abnormal colposcopic findings and comparison of incidences with cytology

The incidence of abnormal findings on colposcopy (ACF), including ACF 1, 2, and 3 was 3.6% (**Figure 1**), and those in women who had undergone vaginal delivery and CS were 1.0 and 2.3%, respectively, whereas that in those who have no history of delivery was 9.8% [7]. Therefore, the screening procedure for women who have no history of delivery should be performed carefully.

In contrast, the incidence of abnormal Pap smear was 1.1%, including incidences of 0.7% (n = 14) for ASC-US, 0.1% (n = 1) for atypical glandular cells (AGC), and 0.3% (n = 6) for low-grade squamous intraepithelial lesion (LSIL). The incidence of abnormal cytology is reasonable for primary screening in Japan.

Note that the incidence of colposcopic abnormality is more frequent than that of cytology.

3. Details of colposcopic abnormality

3.1. Comparison with histology

Abnormal colposcopic findings were compared with histology based on the colposcopy-guided regional biopsies. Women who showed abnormal findings with cytology and/or colposcopy were 2016 in number among those (n = 12,138) who were screened and registered at the Kitasato Gynecologic Tumor Clinic (**Table 1**) [2]. Incidences of benign reparatory lesion, mild, moderate, and severe dysplasia and carcinoma in situ (CIS) were 61.4, 17.1, 7.6, 5.2, and 7.4%, respectively,

Cytology	Histology							
	Benign*	Mild dysplasia	Moderate dysplasia	Severe dysplasia	CIS	Others	Total	No biopsy
NILM	646 (74.6%)	162 (18.7%)	39 (4.5%)	5 (0.6%)	3 (0.3%)	10 (1.2%)	865 (100%)	424
LSIL+HSIL (MD[2*])	124 (52.8%)	46 (19.6%)	28 (11.9%)	26 (11.1%)	5 (2.1%)	6 (2.6%)	235 (100%)	238
ASC	13 (44.8%)	6 (20.7%)	3 (10.3%)	6 (20.7%)		1 (3.4%)	29 (100%)	29
HSIL(SD[3*])	20 (18.5%)	6 (5.6%)	24 (22.2%)	27 (25%)	31 (28.7%)		108 (100%)	8
CIS	4 (10.5%)	3 (7.9%)	4 (10.5%)	1 (2.6%)	26 (68.4%)		38 (100%)	0
SCC	2 (4.8%)	2 (4.8%)	2 (4.8%)	3 (7.1%)	33 (78.6%)		42 (100%)	0
Total	809 (61.4%)	225 (17.1%)	100 (7.6%)	68 (5.2%)	98 (7.4%)	17 (1.3%)	1317 (100%)	699
						Total	2016	

Modified with update in cytologic nomination from Kuramoto et al. [2].

*Squamous metaplasia, reserve cell proliferation and chronic cervicitis.

2*MD=moderate dysplasia.

3*SD=severe dysplasia.

Table 1. Histological diagnosis and cytology in cases with either cytologic or colposcopic abnormality.

among 1317 women who had colposcopy-guided biopsy excluding invasive carcinomas. The benign incidence was 74.6% if cytology ($n = 865$) was negative.

In other words, the majority of histology shows benign lesions, including squamous metaplasia, reserve cell proliferation or chronic cervicitis. We should realize that colposcopic abnormality does not always show neoplastic lesions.

3.2. Abnormal colposcopic findings: extent and characters of the findings

Incidences of abnormal colposcopic findings related to mosaic (M), punctation (P), and aceto-white epithelium (W) are shown in **Table 2**, and those with benign, mild, moderate, and severe dysplasia, CIS, and stage Ia1 were 76.6, 76.6, 80.0, 93.8, and 83.7%, respectively.

Note that the triad of M, P, and W has significant abnormality on the early cervical lesions, including the benign lesions.

The extent of occupying lesions on the vaginal portio were compared with individual SILs, including mild, moderate, and severe dysplasia, and carcinoma *in situ* were compared (**Figure 2**), and the incidences of those >3/4 circle on the portio were 11.4, 8.8, 16.7, and 26.6%, respectively, whereas those of ≤1/4 were 51.6, 40.5, 26.3, and 16.0%, respectively [1].

The abnormal colposcopic area is wider along with the more severe lesion.

The characteristic abnormal findings of colposcopy were the triad of mosaic (M), punctation (P), and aceto-white epithelium (W) (**Figure 3**). When compared with each of SILs, incidences

http://dx.doi.org/10.5772/intechopen.68358

of those of single M, P, or W in mild, moderate, and severe dysplasia, and CIS were 56.0, 54.0, 40.5, and 30.7, whereas those of combined M, P, and W were 33.2, 37.4, 50.0, and 46.4%, respectively, and those of M, P, and W + aV were 4.5, 5.6, 7.0, and 19.2%, respectively [1].

Colposcopic findings \ Diagnosis	benign		mild & moderate dysplasia		Severe dysplasia		CIS		Stage Ia1	
UCF	1 (0.3%)		1 (0.5%)		2 (6.7%)		1 (1.3%)		3 (6.1%)	
NCF	56 (19.0%)		33 (18.0%)		1 (3.3%)		1 (1.3%)		1 (2.0%)	
M.P.W. single	141 (48.1%)		87 (47.6%)		10 (33.3%)		15 (18.7%)		5 (10.2%)	
M.P.W. combined	61 (20.7%)	225 (76.6%)	41 (22.4%)	140 (76.6%)	9 (30.0%)	24 (80.0%)	35 (43.7%)	75 (93.%)	20 (40.9%)	41 (83.7%)
M.P.W.+aV	18 (6.1%)		12 (6.6%)		5 (16.7%)		23 (28.7%)		15 (30.6%)	
M.P.W.+IC	5 (1.7%)						2 (2.5%)		1 (2.0%)	
aV	9 (3.1%)		9 (4.9%)		3 (10.0%)		2 (2.5%)		2 (4.1%)	
IC	3 (1.0%)						1 (1.3%)		2 (4.1%)	
Total	294 (100%)		183 (100%)		30 (100%)		80 (100%)		49 (100%)	

Table 2. Variety of colposcopic findings and cervical lesions.

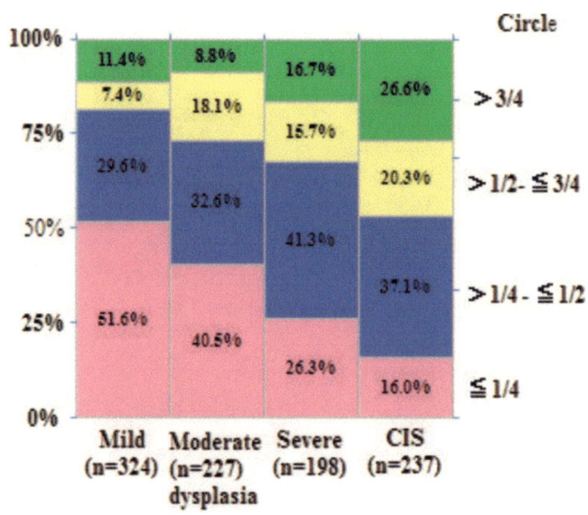

Figure 2. Extent of occupying lesions on abnormality in circle and SILs [1].

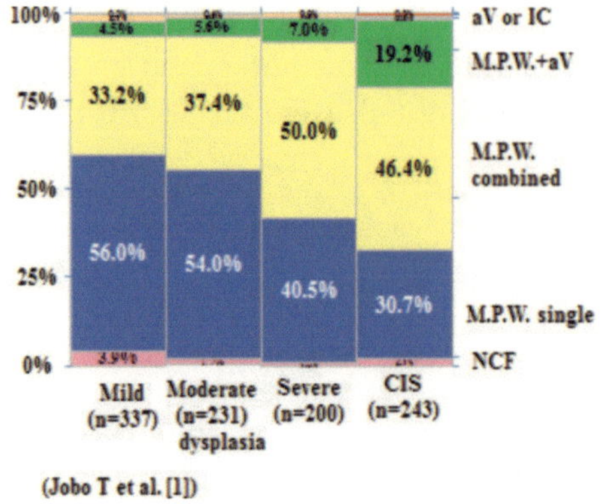

Figure 3. Abnormal findings in colposcopy and SILs [1].

The combined appearance of the triad of MPW with or without atypical vessels (aV) was more frequent in the more severe lesions.

3.3. Comparison between colposcopy and cytology

The incidences between abnormal findings of colposcopy (ACF) and cytology (≥ASC) are compared in SILs. The positive incidences of colposcopy in mild ($n = 225$), moderate ($n = 100$), and severe ($n = 68$) dysplasia, and CIS (98) were 87.6, 88.0, 95.6, and 99.0%, respectively, whereas those of cytology were 28.0, 61.0, 92.6, and 96.9%, respectively (**Figure 4**) [2]. The later study revealed that the negative incidences of mild ($n = 337$) and moderate ($n = 231$) dysplasia were decreased into 57.5 and 24.2%, respectively (**Table 3**) [1].

Note that colposcopy finds constantly the early lesions irrespective of severity. In contrast, cytology is inferior in detecting less severe lesions of mild or moderate dysplasia.

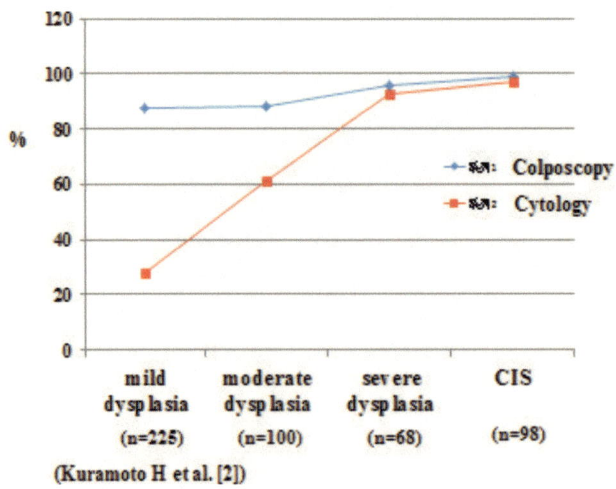

Figure 4. Comparison of abnormal incidences between colposcopy and cytology in SILs [2].

Cytology	Colposcopy	Mild dysplasia (n=337)	Moderate dysplasia (n=231)	Severe dysplasia (n=200)
≥ASC	ACF	130 (38.6%)	171 (74.1%)	176 (88.0%)
	NCF	6 (1.8%)	1 (0.4%)	2 (1.0%)
MLM	ACF	194 (57.5%)	56 (24.2%)	22 (11.0%)
	NCF	7 (2.1%)	3 (1.3%)	0 (0%)

Table 3. Combined effect of cytology and colposcopy [1].

The combined use of cytology and colposcopy, however, is a good combination to elevate the quality of correct diagnosis. In addition, colposcopy fails rarely to find each of mild, moderate, and severe dysplasia being compared with cytology (**Figure 4** and **Table 3**), the results of which show that colposcopy is a good tool for the secondary screening or the detailed examination.

4. Materials and methods

4.1. Materials

4.1.1. For Section 2

The subjects were 1967 consecutive women who underwent screening at the Central Clinic of the Kanagawa Health Service Association using Pap smear and colposcopy simultaneously [7]. The screening programs are based on governmental or company regulations or individual application.

4.1.2. For Section 3

The data are from the registry of Tumor Clinic, Department of Gynecology, Kitasato University Hospital, where the screening for cervix carcinoma was performed by using simultaneous cytology and colposcopy and were analyzed twice at the level of registry numbers (12,138 and 20,900), at which occasion cases who showed abnormal findings either cytology (≥ASC) or colposcopy (≥ACF), excluding invasive carcinoma of the cervix, were 1918 and 2037, respectively.

4.2. Methods of cytology and colposcopy

4.2.1. Pap smear

The cell samples were obtained using a cotton tip (Osaki applicator, Osaki Medical Co. Ltd, Nagoya, Japan) and Cytobrush® plus (Medscand Medical and Cooper Surgical Company, Trumbull, USA) rinsed with physiological saline for the vaginal portio and the cervical canal, respectively, and the cells from the two samples were separately placed onto two slides or each half of a slide, and the tips of the instruments were rotated without making the cell-free area. The slide samples were immediately placed into 95% ethyl alcohol for fixation. Then, the cellular samples were processed using routine Papanicolaou staining procedures.

The cytologic diagnosis for Section 2 was based on the Bethesda System for reporting cervical cytology [8, 9]. The diagnosis for Section 3 was based on the criteria of the Japan Association of Obstetricians and gynecologists (JAOG), which was modified Papanicolaou classification, and rearranged according to the Bethesda System.

4.2.2. Colposcopy

The colposcopic diagnosis was based on the IFCPC 2011 colposcopic classification [10]. Additionally, normal colposcopic findings (NCF) were divided into two subcategories, NCFI and NCFII. Abnormal colposcopic findings (ACF) were divided into three groups, according to their sub-groupings for white epithelium (W), punctation (P), and mosaic (M), which were divided into three categories, as listed below:

1. **NCF**

    1. NCFI: NCF with a squamocolumnar junction (SCJ) localized outside of the external os.

    2. NCFII: NCF with an SCJ localized within the cervical canal that was confirmed by opening the canal with forceps.

2. **ACF**

    1. ACF1: W1, M1, and P1, with which we image squamous metaplasia.

    2. ACF2: W2, M2, and P2, with which we image mild or moderate dysplasia.

    3. ACF3: W3, M3, and P3, with which we image severe dysplasia or carcinoma *in situ*.

    4. ACF4: atypical vessels (aV) associated with W, M, and P, with which microinvasive cancer is suspected.

W was quantitatively subgrouped based on thickness, i.e., color (bluish, pure, or ivory white) and surface texture (smooth or coarse). M was based on the presence of a regular or irregular vessel network and vessel diameter. P was based on the distance between Ps and P shape.

4.2.3. Histology

Colposcopy-guided biopsies, not infrequently multiple, were obtained from the regional ACF areas for histological analysis. SILs were classified into four and adopted the criteria of mild dysplasia, moderate dysplasia, severe dysplasia, or carcinoma *in situ* following Japanese custom, and the most significant portion of diagnosis was selected as the diagnosis of the case.

5. Colposcopy focusing on the lesion in cervical canal

1. Acetic acid is inevitable for colposcopy (**Figures 5–7**).
2. Normal colposcopic findings (NCF) (**Figures 8–10**).
3. Grading of M, P, and W (**Figures 11–13**).
4. Illustrations of colposcopic findings are mandatory (**Figure 14**).
5. Colposcopy-guided "sniping" biopsy taking (**Figure 15**).
6. Special attention on the lesion in cervical canal (**Figures 16–21**).

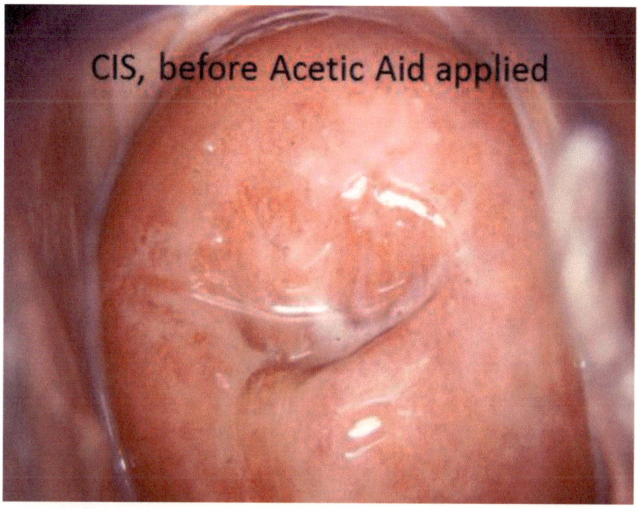

Figure 5. Colposcopic finding before applying acetic acid.

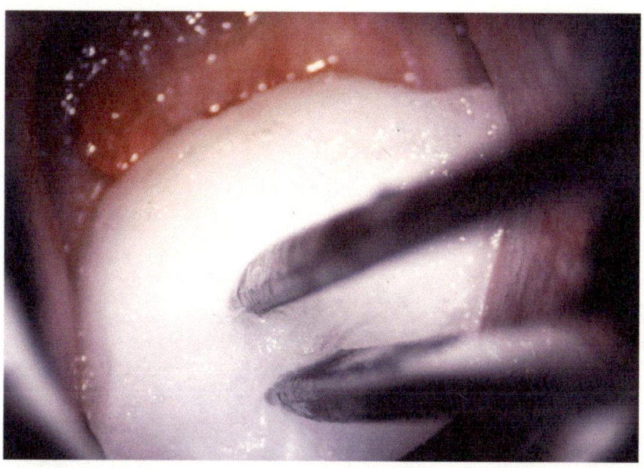

Figure 6. Careful application of 3% acetic acid giving time longer than 30 s is mandatory. A cotton tip being shaped by forceps from cotton ball is effective in the cervical canal.

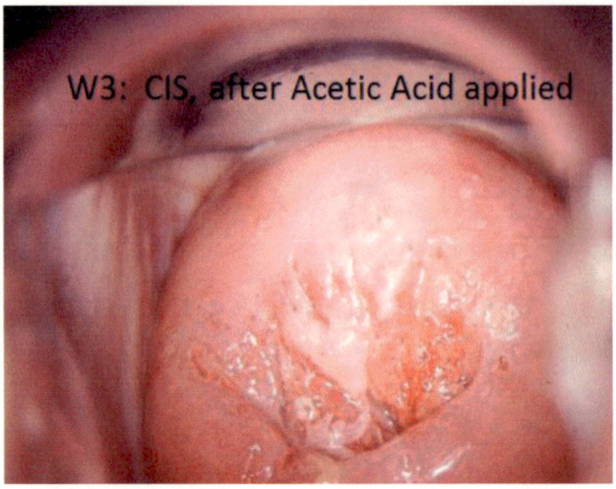

Figure 7. Aceto-white grade 3 (w3) after acetic acid applied.

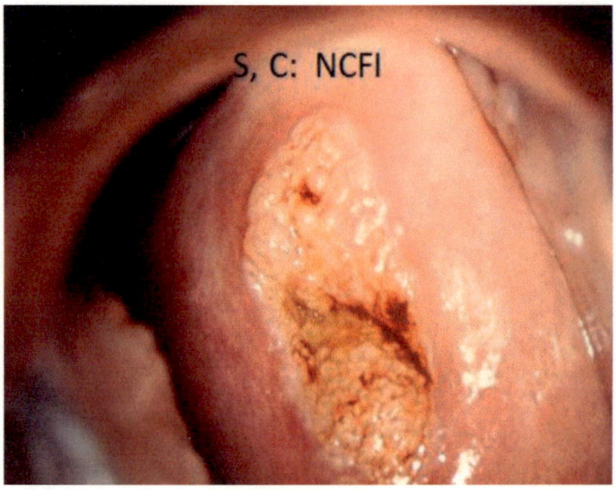

Figure 8. Squamocolumnar junction (SCJ) without transformation zone.

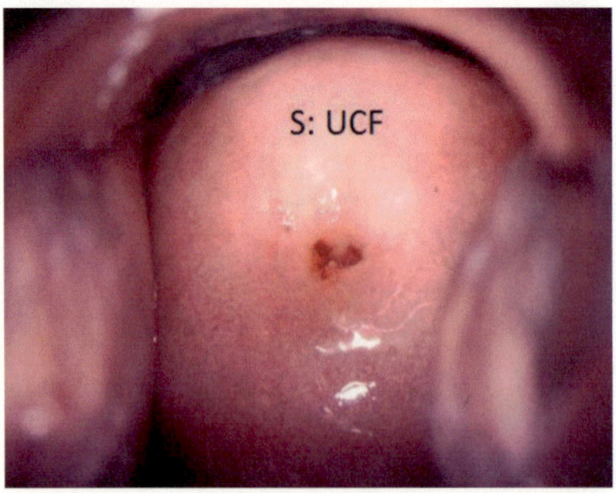

Figure 9. Unsatisfactory colposcopic finding (UCF); SCJ is not visible.

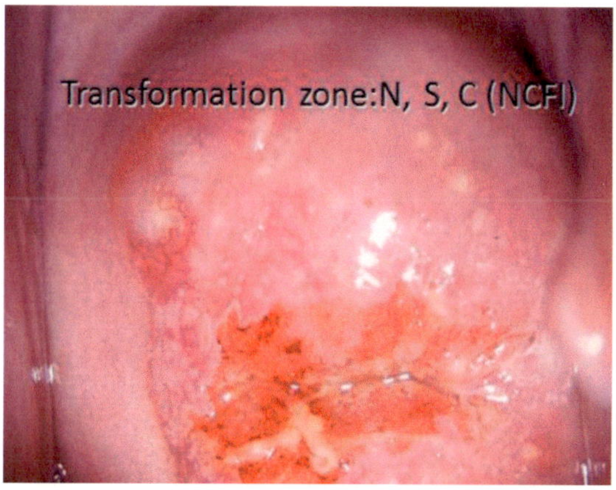

Figure 10. Transformation zone with nabothian follicle.

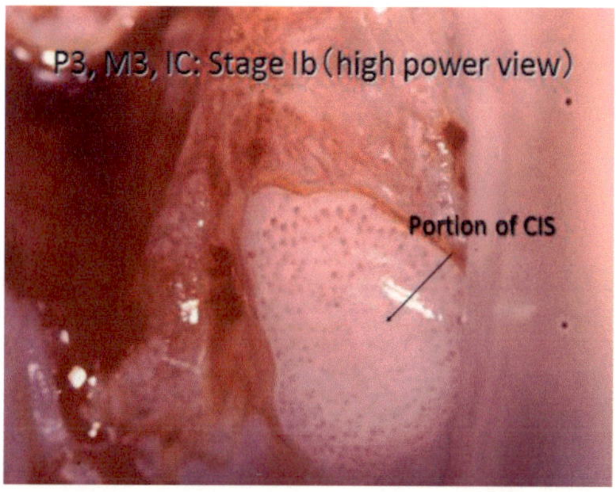

Figure 11. Punctation, grade 3 (P3).

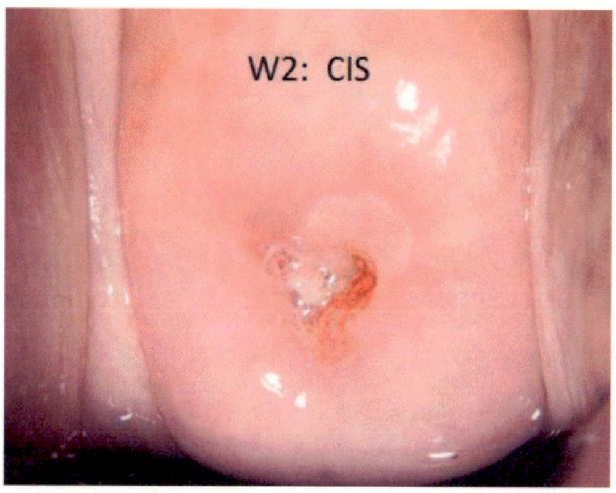

Figure 12. Aceto-white epithelium, grade 2 (W2).

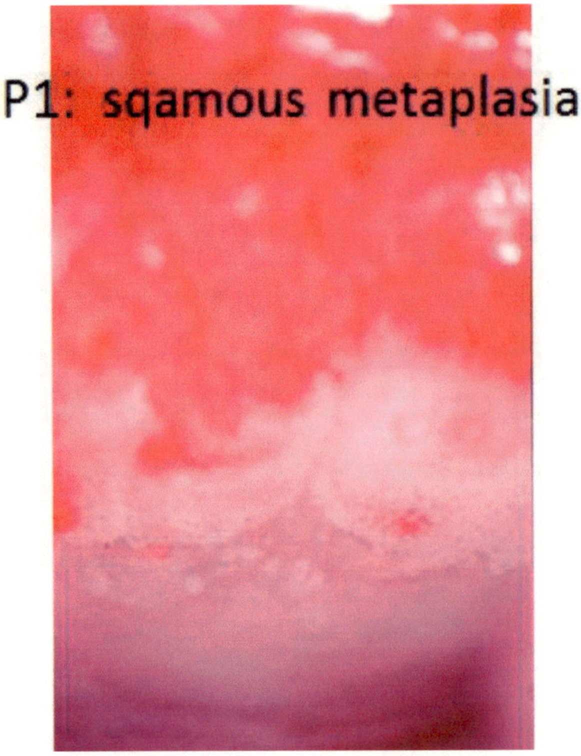

Figure 13. Punctation, grade 1 (P1) of benign lesion.

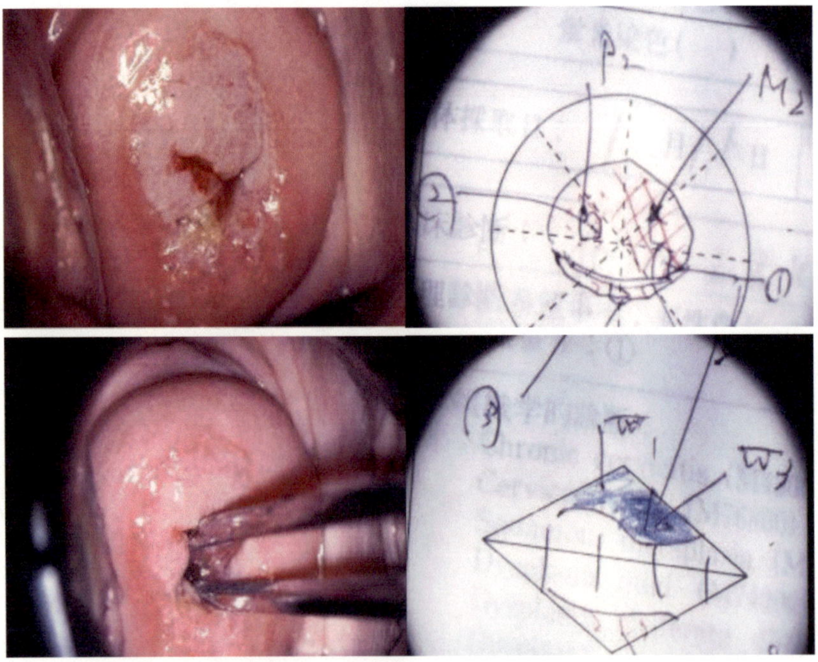

Figure 14. Illustration of colposcopic findings with indicating biopsy points.

http://dx.doi.org/10.5772/intechopen.68358

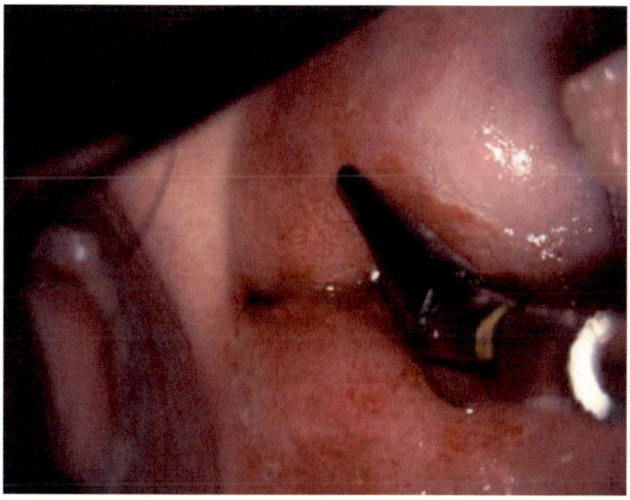

Figure 15. Colposcopy-guided biopsy, being sniped under colposcopic observation.

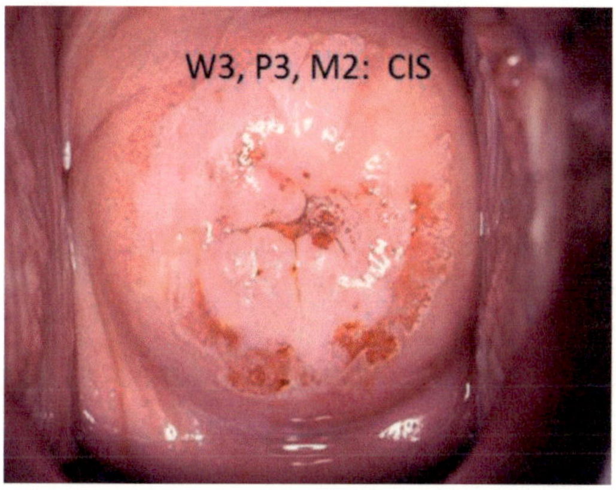

Figure 16. Combined ACFs with a large lesion.

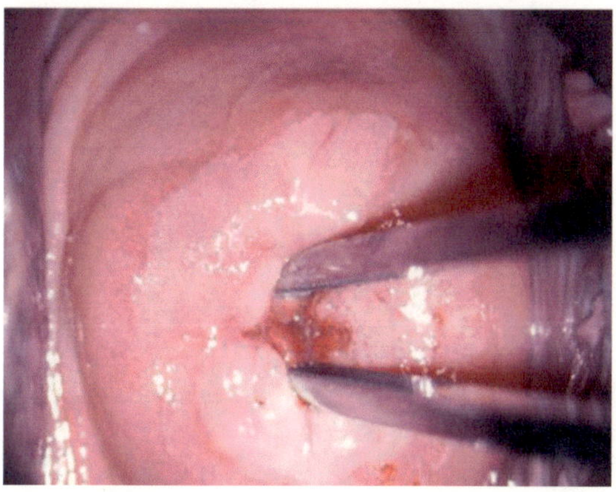

Figure 17. Careful inspection in the cervical canal using a forceps is mandatory.

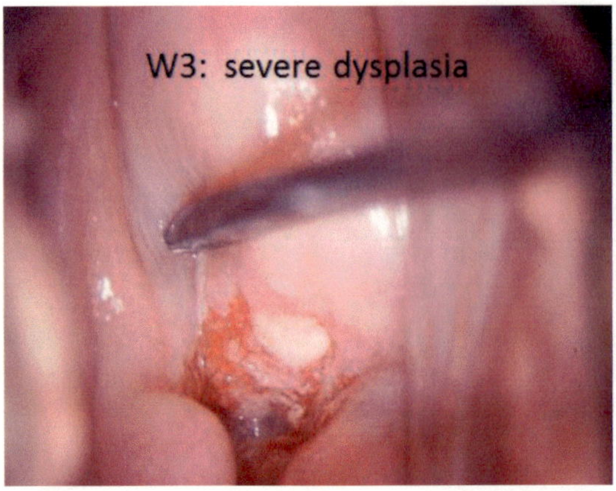

Figure 18. A lesion with W3, localized in the canal.

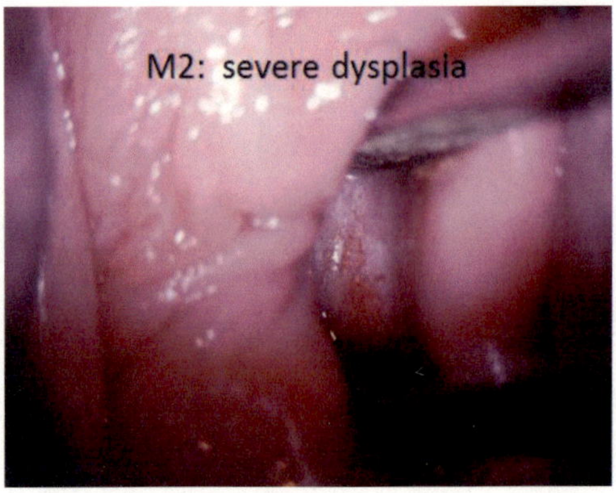

Figure 19. M2 lesion localized in the canal.

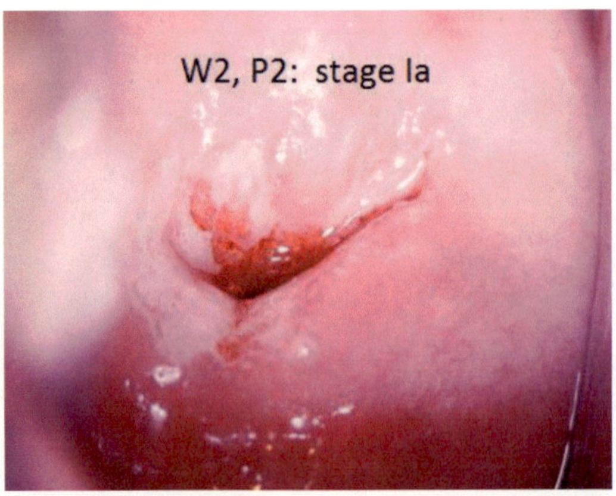

Figure 20. W2 and P2 localized both outside and inside the canal.

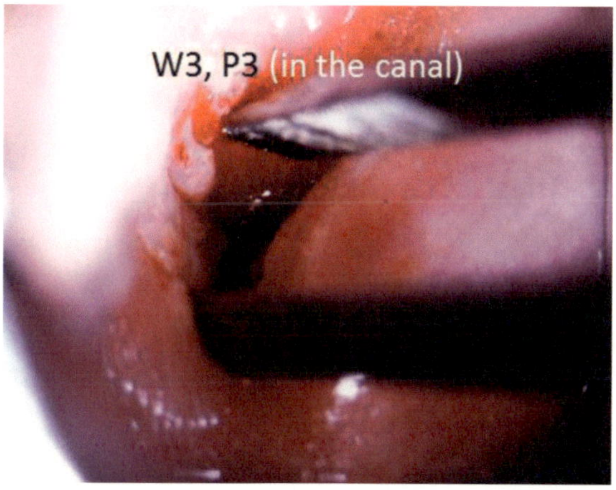

Figure 21. The more significant lesion is located inside the canal.

Author details

Hiroyuki Kuramoto[1,2]* and Toshiko Jobo[3,4]

*Address all correspondence to: kuramoto@yobouigaku-kanagawa.or.jp

1 Department of Cancer Detection for Females, The Kanagawa Health Service Association, Yokohama, Japan

2 Kitasato University, Sagamihara, Japan

3 Gynecologic Oncology Center, (JCHO) Sagamino Hospital, Sagamihara, Japan

4 School of Medicine, Kitasato University, Sagamihara, Japan

References

[1] Jobo T, Wakita K, Sasaki N, Hayashi R, Morisawa T, Tsunoda S, Kuramoto H, Arai M. Diagnosis and treatment of dysplasia of the uterine cervix. Japanese Journal of Cancer & Chemotherapy. 1989;**16**:1592-1597 (in Japanese)

[2] Kuramoto H, Ohno E, Jobo T, Hayashi R. An approach to the diagnosis of dysplasia, CIS and stage Ia cancer using cytology and colposcopy. Obstetrics and Gynecology. 1984;**51**:1289 (in Japanese)

[3] Zur Hausen H. Papillomavirus infection: A major cause of human cancers. Biochemica et Biophysica Acta. 1996;**1288**:F55-F78

[4] Wright TC Jr, Massard LS, Dunton CJ, Spitzer M, Wilkinson EJ, Solomon D. 2006 American Society for Colposcopy and Cervical Pathology-sponsored Consensus Conference. 2006

consensus guidelines for the management of women with cervical intraepithelial neoplasia or adenocarcinoma *in situ*. Journal of Lower Genital Tract Disease. 2007;**11**:223. Erratum in: Journal of Lower Genital Tract Disease.2008;**12**:63

[5] Wight TC Jr. Cervical cancer screening in the 21st century: Is it time to retire the Pap smear? Clinical Obstetrics and Gynecology. 2007;**50**:313

[6] Bosze P. Colposcopy used in a primary setting (routine colposcopy): Advantages and concerns. European Journal of Gynaecological Oncology. 2006;**27**:5

[7] Kuramoto H, Sugimoto N, Iida M. Screening for cancer of the cervix with simultaneous Pap smear and colposcopy. The efficacy of Pap smear and colposcopy. European Journal of Gynaecological Oncology. 2010;**32**:73

[8] Solomon D, Nayar, R, editors. The Bethesda System for Reporting the Cervical Cytology. 2nd ed. New York: Springer; 2004

[9] Japan Society of Obstetricians and Gynecologists (JSOG). Understanding the Reporting Method of Cervical Cytology Based on the Bethesda System. Tokyo, 2008 (in Japanese)

[10] Japan Society of Gynecologic Oncology (JSGO). Revised Standard Atlas of New Colposcopy. Chugai-igaku sha, Tokyo, 2014 (in Japanese)

Section 3

Cervical Pathology

Chapter 6

MiRNAs in Cervical Cancer Radio- and Chemotherapy Response

Jesús Adrián López and
Angelica Judith Granados López

Additional information is available at the end of the chapter

http://dx.doi.org/10.5772/68010

Abstract

Cervical cancer (CC) is a very frequent women disease with high mortality and morbidity incidence worldwide, being the developing countries the most affected. Persistent infection with an oncogenic high-risk human papillomavirus (HPV) type is the primary cause of cervical cancer, but other etiologies are needed for complete malignancy such as patient immune response, genetic, and cellular factors, and/or environment. Radiotherapy in combination with cisplatinum is the standard treatment for invasive cervical cancer. Nevertheless, this conventional treatment is restricted due to eventual development of drug resistance and systemic toxicity. MicroRNAs (miRNAs) are small non-coding RNAs that regulate the expression of protein-coding genes involved in various cellular processes including cancer where they play a very important role in the development and progression of malignancy. As part of this complex disease, miRNAs have been implicated in the process of drug and radiation resistance and sensitivity. Recent studies have been directed to understand how miRNAs under or over-expressed are determinants of clinical response, and other studies have focused to clarify how the process of radio and/or chemotherapy affects miRNA expression. These works could lead to the design of safer and more effective therapy approaches based on miRNA expression and their target regulation.

Keywords: cervical cancer, miRNAs, chemotherapy, radiotherapy

1. Introduction

Cervical cancer (CC) is the third most common malignancy disease worldwide and has the second place in underdeveloped countries [1]. Persistent infection with an oncogenic high-risk human papillomavirus (HPV) is the primary cause of cervical cancer [2], being HR-HPV types 16 and 18 responsible of 95% of cases. However, additional etiologies are needed for complete malignancy to be achieved such as patient immune response, genetic, environmental and/or socioeconomical factors [3, 4]. HPV persistent cell infection could give the opportunity to HPV genome integration [5], which commonly results in viral E2 regulator loss leading to E6 and E7 viral proteins constitutive expression allowing development of dysplasia and malignity [6]. Importantly, HPV integration is frequently found near microRNAs (miRNAs), a type of non-coding RNA genes involved in coding genes post-transcription silencing [7], affecting miRNA expression [8]. Aberrant miRNAs expression has been documented for carcinogenesis development in cervical cancer and several other cancer types [9]. Additionally, miRNA processing machinery misregulation is implicated in carcinogenesis, suggesting that they regulate fundamental processes in cancer progression [10].

Concurrent cisplatin-based chemotherapy added to radiation therapy is the standard treatment for advanced CC. It has been demonstrated that chemotherapy and radiotherapy improve survival rates compared to therapy based on radiation alone or combined hysterectomy and radiation. Although a good response to conventional treatment is achieved by some patients, several global meta-analyses in developed and developing countries have shown that CC patients receiving radiotherapy alone or in combination with different chemotherapeutic agents have at 5 years an overall survival rate from 40 to 70% [11–14]. Additionally, systemic toxicity and side effects are a major problem that patients present during treatment [15]. Therefore, much effort is being made in developing safer and more effective treatment alternatives like natural compounds adjuvants [16–18]. Cisplatin and radiation mechanism of action include damage to DNA and induction of DNA damage response (DDR) that consists of the action of a plethora of genes involved in DNA damage repair. The DDR constitutes the action of detectors of DNA damage, signal transducers and effectors that upon effective action of the DDR proteins the cell will be lead either to survival or apoptosis mechanisms depending on DNA damage severity [19–23]. MiRNAs are active modulators of the DDR mechanisms and have been shown as promoters or inhibitors of radio- and chemosensitivity [24–28]. Additionally, the miRNA response to natural compounds has also been evaluated with respect to treatment resistance and sensitivity [29, 30]. Thus, miRNAs have a clear participation in chemo and radio resistance and sensitivity implying a high potential in gene therapy, prognosis and diagnosis.

2. Cervical cancer etiology

The human papillomavirus (HPV) infection is a common sexual transmission infection associated with cervical intraepithelial neoplasia (CIN) 1, 2, 3, and cervical cancer. More than 80% of women are infected during their life while a just a minority develops malignancy disease [31]. Even though HPV elimination is spontaneous, its persistent cell infection could give the opportunity to HPV genome integration [5] allowing development of dysplasia and malignity [6]. HPV infects mucosa and cutaneous surfaces via cell membrane heparan sulfate proteoglycan [32]. HPV replication is exclusive of the squamous stratified epithelium like epidermis or mucosa membranes of cervix [33]. The genes of HPV are classified in early

(E1, E2, E4, E5, E6, and E7) and late (L1 and L2). The formers are implicated in viral genome replication and transcription, while the latest ones constitute structural virus proteins [34].

Viral genome transcription is dependent on cellular differentiation, specific proteins and RNA profile [35, 36]. Upon HPV infection, viral proteins modify normal cell processes. E4 is related to the delivery of HPV copies from the cell, while E5 is allied in apoptosis resistance [37]. Interaction of E6 with p53 via E6-BP conduces to p53-null phenotype [33, 38] disturbing cell cycle and death [39]. On the other hand, E7 interacts with several proteins to boost G1 to S transition [40–42] permitting cell proliferation, enhancing cancer features [43]. The main cell circuit affected by E7 expression is E2F-Retinoblastoma (E2F-Rb). This oncoprotein binds to Rb liberating E2F transcription factor, promoting the transcription of C-MYC, DNA polymerases, cyclins and CdKs among others [40]. During HPV infection, E2 represses E6 and E7 permitting cell proliferation and differentiation recover. However, in most cervical tumors, E2 is lost during the viral genome integration in the cellular genome allowing, E6 and E7 constitutive expression [6]. It is important to mention that HPV integration is frequently found near miRNA genes [7] affecting miRNA expression [8] and probably some other non-coding RNAs. As it will be mentioned later on, non-coding RNAs, especially micro-RNAs (miRNAs), are important genes in which misregulation is closely linked to cancer development, and therefore, HPV integration is crucial for cervical cancer development [8].

3. MicroRNAs in cervical cancer

MicroRNAs are small non-coding genes that exert their function by silencing of coding genes in almost every cellular process, like, cell proliferation, apoptosis, differentiation, migration, invasion, immune response, and metabolism. Before MiRNAs maturation, pri-miRNAs and pre-miRNAs are sequentially spliced by Drosha and Dicer proteins, respectively, generating a mature 22–24 nucleotides (nt)-long double strand. To perform mRNA silence mature, miRNAs are incorporated into risk silencing complex, and one miRNA strand is lead to base pair to target mRNA [44]. Then, mRNA is degraded after perfect hybridization is achieved or protein translation is inhibited in incomplete base pair hybridization. Aberrant miRNAs expression has been documented for several carcinomas such as breast, cervical, lung, kidney and colon carcinomas among many others [9], and it has been evaluated by microarray, sequencing, northern blotting, cloning, and reverse transcription-polymerase chain reaction (RT-PCR) techniques [45, 46]. Pioneer study relating miRNAs and cervical cancer was made in 2007. In this chapter, they sequenced 166 miRNAs comparing normal tissue, cell lines and tumor tissues, founding six miRNAs with differential expressions. MiR-21 was over-expressed in cell lines and tumor tissue compared with normal tissue, while let-7b, let7-c, miR-23b, miR-143, and miR-196b expressions were reduced [47]. Since then, many studies have addressed the importance of microRNAs in cervical cancer. Confirmation of various works has provided very useful miRNA expression information to study more profoundly the function and application of this miRNAs in cancer therapy, prognosis, and diagnosis. For example, miR-218 has been found down-regulated in cervical cancer tissue, and its low expression has been related to cancer progression, while its up-regulation in Hela cells has shown that it improves cisplatin sensitivity [48–51]. In silico and in vitro studies have shown that miRNAs can potentially regulate more than 100 genes, suggesting a great potential for coding genes regulation in cancer cells [52].

4. Cervical cancer therapy

Concurrent cisplatin-based chemotherapy added to radiation therapy is the standard treatment for locally advanced CC (LACC). It has been demonstrated that chemotherapy and radiotherapy improve survival rates compared to therapy based on radiation alone or combined hysterectomy and radiation. In addition, randomized trials demonstrated improved treatment outcome with combinations of cisplatin and 5-fluorouracil compared with radiation therapy alone. It is established that concurrent chemotherapy increases the severity of acute side effects; however, it does not appear to increase the risk of late side effects of radiotherapy. Although a good response to conventional treatment is achieved by some patients, LACC patients treated with radiotherapy have in general a 50% chance of recurrence or persistent disease. Moreover, several global meta-analyses, including patients treated in developed and developing countries, have shown that CC patients receiving radiotherapy alone or in combination with different chemotherapeutic agents have at 5 years an overall survival rate from 40 to 70% [11–13]. This conventional treatment is restricted due to eventual development of drug resistance and systemic toxicity; therefore, much effort is being made in developing safer and effective alternatives like natural compounds as anti-cancer drugs [16–18].

Other approaches have been made toward developing cisplatin analogues with improved chemotherapeutic efficacy and reduced toxic side effects, the most notable of these being carboplatin and oxaliplatin clinically registered [53]. Individual trials have suggested that other drugs, including mitomycin and epirubicin, might be beneficial [54]. It has been investigated the administration of neoadjuvant chemotherapy (NAC), which includes cisplatin, paclitaxel, and carboplatin after radiation therapy enhancing the treatment response [55]. Although the evidence for benefit of concurrent chemotherapy is strong for newly diagnosed, loco-regionally advanced cervical cancers confined to the pelvis, the relative benefits and risks are not well understood for patients who require larger fields of radiotherapy [54]. Many studies are currently being made to improve CC cancer treatment for a major patient percent recovery and less side effects by different approaches as miRNA-based therapy.

5. Cisplatin action mechanism

DNA is vulnerable to damage that originates from endogenous metabolites, such as macrophages and neutrophils produced reactive oxygen species (ROS), reactive nitrogen species (RNS) [56] and exogenous agents including smoking, chemical carcinogens, radiation [57], and genotoxic cancer therapeutics [58]. For instance, cisplatin, cis-diamminedichloroplatinum

(II) (NH3)2PtCl2) is a DNA-damaging agent used extensively as a chemotherapeutic drug. Particularly, it is successfully employed to treat different cancer types like ovarian and testicular carcinomas, as well as a range of other solid tumors [59, 60]. However, dose-limiting toxic side effects and the occurrence of both acquired and intrinsic drug resistance in cells impose great limitations on cisplatin chemotherapy [61–63].

A hallmark of cisplatin toxicity is loss of outer hair-cells (OHCs) beginning from the cochlear base. A recent study suggests additionally the involvement of stria vascularis and spiral ganglion [64]. One-third of cisplatin-treated cancer patients develop irreversible hearing loss [15]. It has been demonstrated that the toxic side effects of cisplatin depend on the drug cell transportation via the copper transporter CTR1, previously implicated in cisplatin-induced nephrotoxicity [65, 66] or the organic cation transporter OCT2. Upon partial solvolization, cisplatin forms $[(NH_3)_2PtCl(H_2O)]+$ (monoaqua complex), which can be transported by OC.

Although cisplatin detailed mechanism of action is presently unclear, it is generally thought that the covalent binding of cisplatin to cellular DNA and subsequent formation of bulky platinum-DNA (Pt-DNA) adducts mediates the cytotoxicity of this anti-cancer agent [67, 68]. Intra-strand DNA cross-links are the most common adducts formed, although inter-strand DNA cross-links and DNA-protein cross-links can also occur [69, 70]. The intra-strand DNA lesions preferentially form between the N-7 of adjacent guanine residues, inhibiting the passage of polymerases and thus interfering with DNA replication and RNA transcription inside target cells [71–74].

The active response to cisplatin induces DNA damage entailing two key processes. (1) Repair of DNA damage through the removal of cisplatin adducts and (2) induction of cell death via apoptosis when repair cannot be carried out successfully. Among these DNA repair pathways, NER repairs damaged DNA commonly caused by chemotherapeutics such as platinum drugs, which has been proven to be associated with chemotherapy resistance in non-small cell lung cancer (NSCLC) [19].

Cisplatin's mechanism of action in addition to cell cycle arrest and apoptosis includes cellular senescence through activation of onco-suppressing p53 and p16 proteins, and there is strong evidence that p53 plays a role in cisplatin sensitivity [75]. Transcription factor NFκB and the serine/threonine kinase Akt play critical roles in cancer cell survival and have been shown to be activated in various malignancies [76]. Thus, efforts are underway to identify alternate therapies, including the use of curcumin in combination with radiation and/or chemotherapeutic drugs in hepatic, ovarian, and head and neck squamous cell cancer HNSCC [77–79]. It is believed that the therapeutic potential of cisplatin will be enhanced with the addition of curcumin, with lower, less toxic doses of cisplatin required for its cytotoxic effect [30].

6. Ionizing radiation action mechanism

Ionizing radiation is a type of high-energy radiation that in contact with atoms and molecules releases electrons generating ions that can break covalent bonds. Ionizing radiation directly affects DNA structure by inducing DNA breaks, particularly double-strand breaks (DSBs). Secondary effects are the generation of reactive oxygen species (ROS) that oxidize proteins and lipids and induce several damages to DNA like generation of a basic sites and single-strand breaks (SSBs). Quiescent and slowly dividing cells are less radiosensitive, like those constituting the nervous system, while cells with high proliferation rates are more radiosensitive, like bone marrow, skin, and epithelial cells of the gastro-intestinal tract, among others. Ionizing radiation can be divided into X-rays, gamma rays, alpha, and beta particles, and neutrons. The radiation dose is measured in gray (Gy) units, a measure of the amount of radiation absorbed by 1 kg of tissue [20].

Radiotherapy is a treatment aimed at shrinking the tumor mass or at eliminating residual tumor cells by exposing the tumor to ionizing radiation. Radiotherapy regimes mostly use X- and gamma radiation and affect tumor and healthy irradiated cells indistinctly [80].

Ionizing radiation causes DSBs directly, and reactive oxygen species (ROS) caused by radiation also indirectly damages DNA. ROS generate apurinic/apyrimidinic (abasic) sites in the DNA, SSBs, sugar moiety modifications, and deaminated adducted bases [81, 82]. After DNA damage, the cell repair machinery is activated and stops the cell cycle at specific control checkpoints to prevent continuation of the cycle and repair damaged DNA. If tumor cells can efficiently repair the radiation damage, resistance to radiation develops, enabling cells to survive and replicate. If the damage remains unrepaired, these mechanisms induce programmed cell death or apoptosis to prevent accumulation of mutations in daughter cells [83, 84]. Ionizing radiation unavoidably spreads to normal tissue, inducing side effects in tumor-adjacent normal cells that may contribute to chromosomal aberrations and to increase the risk for new malignancies. Therefore, reduced patients survival could be a consequence of high radiation doses administation [21].

Individual radiation treatment based on DSB repair capability could predict toxicity to surrounding tissues, thereby improving treatment safety. DSB repair capability depends not just on gene integrity, but also on gene expression. For example, genetic and epigenetic mechanisms may reduce or abrogate the expression of genes involved in DSB repair [85]. DNA repair is orchestrated by a series of pathways, mainly including nucleotide excision repair (NER), base excision repair (BER), DNA mismatch repair (MMR), and single-strand break repair (SSBs) [86]. DSB repair is achieved in three ways: non-homologous end joining (NHEJ), conservative homologous recombination (HR), and single-strand alignment (SSA), also called non-conservative homologous recombination [87].

Three interconnected sensor systems have been described that have the ability to detect a single DSB within minutes after its formation [88]: (1) PI3K-related kinases (PIKKs), (2) ataxia telangiectasia and Rad3-related (ATR), ataxia telangiectasia mutated (ATM) and (3) DNA-dependent protein kinase (DNA-PK). ATR participates in the recognition of SSBs induced by cisplatin or IR, whereas ATM is essentially implicated DSBs recognition. Importantly, damage signals are transduced to the cell, while cells react to decide to either repair damaged DNA or activate cell cycle checkpoints or induce apoptosis. Upon DSBs induced by cisplatin and/or radiation, as a transducer, the targets of ATM/ATR with dual-functions promote survival or cell death. Meanwhile, cell signaling pathways activate cell cycle checkpoint halting its progression proving time to cells to repair the damage by the recruitment of DNA repair proteins to facilitate DSB repair triggered by NHEJ or HR, depending on the cell cycle phase [22]. If DNA damage is greater than the repair capacity, hence replication and transcription will be blocked, and DDR signals activate downstream cell death pathways. Importantly, DNA repair genes are actively regulated by miRNAs, which are highly found misregulated in cervical cancer and have marked effect on chemo- and radiotherapy resistance, implying a big target potential in gene therapy.

7. MiRNAs in mechanisms of cancer therapy resistance

Some studies have enlightened miRNAs contribution to chemo- and radiotherapy response; for example, it was shown that cisplatin, paclitaxel, and carboplatin prior to laparoscopic radical hysterectomy (LRH) improved patient response by inducing p53, miR-34a, and miR-605 expression, while levels of E2F1 and Mdm2 were significantly low [55]. Additionally, alternative less toxic natural compounds are analyzed; for example, it was shown that I′5-I′acetoxichavicol acetate (ACA) induced comparable levels of dose- and time-dependent cytotoxicity on a variety of tumor cell lines to current commercial anticancer drugs, without any adverse effects on normal cells [29]. A total of 25 miRNAs were found to be expressed significantly different in response to ACA and/or cisplatin including has-miR-138, has-miR-210, has-miR-744 which target genes involved in apoptosis and cell cycle progression regulating pathways [89].

Genotoxic agents, such as UV light, γ-irradiation, oxidative stress, and chemical mutagens, induce a DDR that results in the up- and down-regulation of miRNAs expression levels that will happen in a few hours after DNA damage and will return to basal levels in 24 h. MiRNA DDR seems to be influenced by type of damaging agent, radiation Gy dose and time of exposure as well as cell type involved [90–94]. MiRNA-induced response has been documented as transcriptionally modulated miRNA expression and biogenesis modulation miRNA maturation.

In response to DNA damage, the ATM or ATR kinase activates p53, which in turn transactivates genes involved in cell cycle regulation, senescence, and apoptosis. A clear example is the transactivation of miRNA-34 family by p53 upon DNA damage and oncogenic stress [95]. MiR-34a ectopic expression leads to G1 phase cell cycle arrest in both primary and tumor-derived cell lines likely through silencing a program of genes that promote cell cycle progression. In addition to the miR-34 family, miR-192, miR-194, miR-215, and miR-17-92 cluster are other miRNAs found to be transcriptionally regulated by p53. In addition, other DNA damage responsive transcription factors, such as NF-κB, c-Myc, CREB and E2F1, modulate miRNA expression [96, 97]. However, the specific functions of those miRNAs in DNA damage need further study.

MiRNAs involvement in DDR seems to be additionally modulated beyond transcription regulation by transcription factors through post-transcription modulation. Miyazono group′s study demonstrated that several miRNAs, including miR-16-1, miR-143 and miR-145, were post-transcriptionally up-regulated in a p53-dependent and p68/p72-dependent manner upon genotoxic stress [98, 99]. In colorectal HCT116 and lung WI-38 cell lines, p53 interacts with the Drosha processing complex through direct interaction with p68 and, in turn, facilitates the processing of primiRNAs to pre-miRNAs. Apparently, the guardians of genome, p53/p63/p73, modulate the processing of a group of miRNAs, including the tumor suppressor miRNAs, let-7, miR-34, miR-15/16a, miR-145, miR-26, miR-29, and miR-146a [100]. Another protein modulating miRNA processing is KSRP, a KH type splicing ribonucleoprotein that serves as a critical component of both Drosha and Dicer complexes and regulates the biogenesis of a subset of miRNAs like miR-16 and miR-143 and miR-145 by Drosha and Dicer respectively [101].

As a response to DNA damage, a novel class of small RNAs, named DDR-regulating RNAs (DDRNAs), has been identified near double-strand breaks (DSB) [102]. It has also been reported the presence of Dicer-dependent small RNAs (named DSB-induced RNAs, diRNAs) arising from the sequences flanking DSBs in plants and in human cells [103]. At the moment how do these site-specific small RNAs act to control DDR activation, it is not clear; however, it seems that the presence of DSB-derived site-specific small RNAs may be a universal phenomenon in DNA damage, involved in recruitment of chromatin-modifying complexes to sites of damage or guiding DNA repair signaling [104].

MiRNAs are also involved in mechanisms of multidrug resistance (MDR) like dysregulation of drugs transporters, defects of apoptosis and autophagy machinery, alterations of drug metabolism and drug targets, and disruption of redox homeostasis [28]. Some miRNAs regulating drug transporters like (P-gp/ABCB)1 are miR-451, miR-27a [105–108], miR-138 [109], miR-298 [110], miR-381, and miR-495 [111]. The entire process of autophagy, including autophagic induction, vesicle nucleation, vesicle elongation, and completion, can be modulated by different miRNAs [28]. Some miRNAs documented in this cellular process are miR-30a [112], miR-30d [113], miR-204 [114], miR-16 and miR-17 [115, 116], miR-200b, miR-15a [116], and miR-181a [117]. Metabolic regulation by miRNAs has been documented for miR-27b, which can modulate resistance to docetaxel in cancerous cells [118, 119] and sensitizes cancer cells to a broad spectrum of anti-cancer drugs in vitro and in vivo by activating P53-dependent apoptosis and reducing CYP1B1-mediated drug detoxification [120], and for miR-892a that targets CYP1A1 [121]. Apparently, miRNAs can impact anti-cancer drugs sensitivity by modulating the expression of drug targets. For example, miR-192 and miR-215 may influence 5-FU sensitivity by targeting Tynidilate synthetase (TS) enzyme in colorectal cancer cells [122], while miR-211 can increase the sensitivity of pancreatic cancer cells to gemcitabine [123], and let-7 negatively regulates RRM2 expression and sensitizes PDAC cells to gemcitabine [28].

8. MicroRNAs in cervical cancer chemo- and radiotherapy resistance

Additionally to several works involving coding genes, other efforts involving miRNAs are being made for the understanding of cellular chemo- and radiosensitivity. In this context, it has been shown that miRNAs expression is affected in radio and chemo-resistant cells [25–28]. Some miRNAs have been identified as promoters of radioresistance such as miR-421, which regulates the activity of DNA repair ATM protein [124]; miR-23b and miR-34a, which are regulated by p53 protein [125]; miR-106b, which silences cell cycle regulator protein p21 and promotes cell cycle progression and overrides a doxorubicin-induced DNA damage checkpoint and miR-17-92 cluster [126, 127]; while others have been found as radiosensitizers such as miR-424 promoting radiosensitivity by targeting aprataxin, which stimulates DNA repair and protects cells against genotoxic stress in cancer cells [128] and miR-375 promoting radiosensitivity of HR-HPV-positive cervical cancer cells by targeting the ubiquitin ligase mRNA (UBE3A) leading to decreased p53 degradation and thereby increasing radiation-induced apoptosis [129]. Interestingly, miR-375 was also found increased in acquired paclitaxel resistance in cervical cancer [130].

Some studies have shown that miRNAs involved in chemosensitivy promotion. For instance, the sensitivity to cisplatin is augmented via miR-181a Protein Kinase C Delta (PRKCD) silencing [131] and miR-218, which also impairs tumor growth and induces apoptosis via AKT-mTOR pathway in HeLa cells [50]. Additionally, miR-218 enhances Rapamacyn sensitivity by mTor pathway Rictor targeting [132]. An study showed that p53:miR-34a:E2F1 and p53:miR-605:Mdm2 are activated after chemotherapy with cisplatin, paclitaxel, and carboplatin cycles improving the treatment response of cervical cancer patients [55]. Other cisplatin sensitizing miRNAs are miR-15b and miR-16 that target Bcl2 in Hela cells [133], while miR-15a and miR-16 induce autophagy and sensitize cells to camptothecin [116]. Other miRNAs promote chemosensitivity to other drugs, for example, miR-126 additionally to hinder proliferation it enhances sensitivity to bleomycin [134]; mir-125a, promotes paclitaxel sensitivity via silencing of signal transducer and activator of transcription (STAT3) [135], and miR-145 that is regulated by p53 influences sensitivity to mitomycin and reverses the chemoresistance induced by glucocorticoids [136].

Recent works have focused on the design of radio and chemotherapy response predictors. Pedroza-Torres and cols identified a miRNA expression signature based on the over-expression of seven miRNAs (miR-31-3p, miR-3676, miR-125a-5p, miR-100-5p, miR-125b-5p, miR-200a-5p, and miR-342) to identify CC patients who could fail to conventional, treatment based on chemo- and radiotherapy [137]. Other works have provided similar valuable information, for example, miR-200a and miR-9 signature could predict patient survival. Particularly, miR-200a could affect the metastatic potential of cancer cells by negatively regulating cell motility genes [138]. Another study indicated that the miRNA signature consisting of miR-630, miR-1246, miR-1290, and miR-3138 could promote radio resistance of CC cells [138–140].

A total of 25 miRNAs were found to be differentially expressed in response to 1S-1-acetoxychavicol acetate (ACA) and/or cisplatin. MiR-138, miR-210, and miR-744 have predicted gene targets involved in signaling pathways regulating apoptosis and cell cycle progression. Remarkable, ACA acts as a chemosensitizer that synergistically potentiates the cytotoxic effect of cisplatin in cervical cancer cells. MiRNA expression changes with the administration of ACA and/or cisplatin suggests that miRNAs play an important role in anticancer drug responses making them ideal for therapeutic treatment of patients with chemoresistance [89].

Curcumin (Cur) is a phenolic compound purified from the rhizome of Curcuma longa, historically used in traditional medicine [141, 142]. It has been reported that Cur reduces the expression and function of P-glycoprotein (P-gp), a protein highly expressed in tumoral cells [143]. This natural compound and derivatives have been catalogued as not toxic in humans even at high doses (12 g/day) [144]. Cur efficacy is limited due to the low level of oral bioavailability, poor absorption ability, a high metabolic rate, inactivity of metabolic products, rapid elimination and clearance from the body, poor pharmacokinetics and solubility, and degradation under natural to basic pH conditions. Conjugation of Cur to nanoparticles (NPs) and anti-P-glycoprotein (P-gp) antibody (Cur-NPs-APgp) targeting to P-gp could enhance paclitaxel (PTX) sensitivity both in vitro and in vivo [140]. Curcumin reverses cisplatin resistance in SiHa-resistant phenotype (SiHaR) cells by overcoming over-expression of multidrug resistance protein 1 (MRP1) and Pgp1 and sensitized cervical cancer cells toward cisplatin-induced cell killing with lower chemotherapeutic drug dose [145]. Recent evidence has suggested curcumin-induced modulation of the expression of several miRNAs such as suppression of oncomiRs miR-21, miR-17-5p, miR-20a, and miR-27a and over-expression of miR-34 a/c and epithelial-mesenchymal transition-suppressor miRNAs among the most important effects of curcumin on miRNA homeostasis [24].

Other natural compounds with anticancer potential are Cratoxylum formosum subsp. pruniflorum (Kurz.) Gogel. (Teawdang) phenolic extracts that could inhibit growth of HeLa and Siha cancer cell lines [146]. Teawdang is a northeast Thai vegetable that contains several bioactive constituents especially chlorogenic acid which has radical scavenging activity [147]. Thus, miRNA regulation investigation of these bioactive compounds is recommended. It could be very supportive the study of miRNA response to other natural compounds with anticancer potential and drug resistance overcome like Chrysin from Thai propolis [148]; a series of ferrocene and (arene)ruthenium(II) complexes attached to the naturally occurring anticancer naphthoquinones plumbagin and juglone [149]; sesquiterpene lactones isolated from Illicium simonsii [150]; phenanthroindolizidine alkaloids, (−)-(R)-13aalpha-antofine (1) and (−)-(R)-13aalpha-6-O-desmethylantofine (2) and natural products, (−)-(R)-13a alpha-secoantofine (3) and (−)-(R)-13a alpha-6-O-desmethylsecoantofine isolated from Cynanchum vincetoxicum [151].

9. Conclusions and considerations

In the present literature, it is reviewed, analyzed, and organized novel information regarding miRNAs involved in resistance to drugs, natural compounds and radiation in cervical cancer treatment. The present data could encourage future research to generate optimal treatment strategies for individual patients especially before the course of chemo- and radiotherapy based on miRNAs regulation, conventional and non-conventional cervical cancer therapy.

Author details

Jesús Adrián López[1,2] and Angelica Judith Granados López[1,2]*

*Address all correspondence to: agranadosjudith@gmail.com

1 Laboratory of microRNAs, Academic Unit of Biological Sciences, Autonomic University of Zacatecas, Zacatecas, Mexico

2 Doctorate in Basic Sciences, Area of Basic Sciences, Autonomic University of Zacatecas, Zacatecas, México.

References

[1] Jemal, A., et al., Global cancer statistics. CA Cancer J Clin, 2011. **61**(2): pp. 69-90.

[2] Walboomers, J.M., et al., Human papillomavirus is a necessary cause of invasive cervical cancer worldwide. J Pathol, 1999. **189**(1): pp. 12-9.

[3] Haverkos, H., M. Rohrer, and W. Pickworth., The cause of invasive cervical cancer could be multifactorial. Biomed Pharmacother, 2000. **54**(1): pp. 54-9.

[4] Perez-Plasencia, C., A. Duenas-Gonzalez, and B. Alatorre-Tavera, Second hit in cervical carcinogenesis process: involvement of wnt/beta catenin pathway. Int Arch Med, 2008. **1**(1): p. 10.

[5] Melnikow, J., et al., Natural history of cervical squamous intraepithelial lesions: a meta-analysis. Obstet Gynecol, 1998. **92**(4 Pt 2): pp. 727-35.

[6] Arias-Pulido, H., et al., Human papillomavirus type 16 integration in cervical carcinoma in situ and in invasive cervical cancer. J Clin Microbiol, 2006. **44**(5): pp. 1755-62.

[7] Calin, G.A., et al., Human microRNA genes are frequently located at fragile sites and genomic regions involved in cancers. Proc Natl Acad Sci U S A, 2004. **101**(9): p. 2999-3004.

[8] Granados Lopez, A.J. and J.A. Lopez, Multistep model of cervical cancer: participation of miRNAs and coding genes. Int J Mol Sci, 2014. **15**(9): pp. 15700-33.

[9] Kumar, M.S., et al., Impaired microRNA processing enhances cellular transformation and tumorigenesis. Nat Genet, 2007. **39**(5): pp. 673-7.

[10] Muralidhar, B., et al., Functional evidence that Drosha overexpression in cervical squamous cell carcinoma affects cell phenotype and microRNA profiles. J Pathol, 2011. **224**(4): pp. 496-507.

[11] Chemoradiotherapy for Cervical Cancer Meta-Analysis, C., Reducing uncertainties about the effects of chemoradiotherapy for cervical cancer: a systematic review and

meta-analysis of individual patient data from 18 randomized trials. J Clin Oncol, 2008. **26**(35): pp. 5802-12.

[12] Hart, K., et al., Postoperative radiation for cervical cancer with pathologic risk factors. Int J Radiat Oncol Biol Phys, 1997. **37**(4): pp. 833-8.

[13] Keys, H. and S.K. Gibbons, *Optimal management of locally advanced cervical carcinoma.* J Natl Cancer Inst Monogr, 1996(21): pp. 89-92.

[14] Delaney, G., et al., The role of radiotherapy in cancer treatment: estimating optimal utilization from a review of evidence-based clinical guidelines. Cancer, 2005. **104**(6): pp. 1129-37.

[15] Li, Y., R.B. Womer, and J.H. Silber, Predicting cisplatin ototoxicity in children: the influence of age and the cumulative dose. Eur J Cancer, 2004. **40**(16): pp. 2445-51.

[16] Zaman, M.S., et al., Curcumin nanoformulation for cervical cancer treatment. Sci Rep, 2016. **6**: p. 20051.

[17] Prusty, B.K. and B.C. Das, Constitutive activation of transcription factor AP-1 in cervical cancer and suppression of human papillomavirus (HPV) transcription and AP-1 activity in HeLa cells by curcumin. Int J Cancer, 2005. **113**(6): pp. 951-60.

[18] Di Domenico, F., et al., Antioxidants in cervical cancer: chemopreventive and chemotherapeutic effects of polyphenols. Biochim Biophys Acta, 2012. **1822**(5): pp. 737-47.

[19] Rosell, R., et al., Nucleotide excision repair pathways involved in Cisplatin resistance in non-small-cell lung cancer. Cancer Control, 2003. **10**(4): pp. 297-305.

[20] Hawley, L., Principles of radiotherapy. Br J Hosp Med (Lond), 2013. **74**(11): pp. C166-9.

[21] Brown, L.C., R.W. Mutter, and M.Y. Halyard, Benefits, risks, and safety of external beam radiation therapy for breast cancer. Int J Womens Health, 2015. **7**: pp. 449-58.

[22] Helleday, T., et al., DNA repair pathways as targets for cancer therapy. Nat Rev Cancer, 2008. **8**(3): pp. 193-204.

[23] Christmann, M. and B. Kaina, Transcriptional regulation of human DNA repair genes following genotoxic stress: trigger mechanisms, inducible responses and genotoxic adaptation. Nucleic Acids Res, 2013. **41**(18): pp. 8403-20.

[24] Momtazi, A.A., et al., Curcumin as a MicroRNA regulator in cancer: a review. Rev Physiol Biochem Pharmacol, 2016. **171**: pp. 1-38.

[25] Kitahara, O., et al., Classification of sensitivity or resistance of cervical cancers to ionizing radiation according to expression profiles of 62 genes selected by cDNA microarray analysis. Neoplasia, 2002. **4**(4): pp. 295-303.

[26] Tewari, D., et al., Gene expression profiling of in vitro radiation resistance in cervical carcinoma: a feasibility study. Gynecol Oncol, 2005. **99**(1): pp. 84-91.

[27] Wong, Y.F., et al., Expression genomics of cervical cancer: molecular classification and prediction of radiotherapy response by DNA microarray. Clin Cancer Res, 2003. **9**(15): pp. 5486-92.

[28] An, X., et al., Regulation of multidrug resistance by microRNAs in anti-cancer therapy. Acta Pharm Sin B, 2017. **7**(1): pp. 38-51.

[29] Awang, K., et al., The apoptotic effect of 1′s-1′-acetoxychavicol acetate from Alpinia conchigera on human cancer cells. Molecules, 2010. **15**(11): pp. 8048-59.

[30] Duarte, V.M., et al., Curcumin enhances the effect of cisplatin in suppression of head and neck squamous cell carcinoma via inhibition of IKKbeta protein of the NFkappaB pathway. Mol Cancer Ther, 2010. **9**(10): pp. 2665-75.

[31] Scheurer, M.E., G. Tortolero-Luna, and K. Adler-Storthz, Human papillomavirus infection: biology, epidemiology, and prevention. Int J Gynecol Cancer, 2005. **15**(5): pp. 727-46.

[32] Giroglou, T., et al., Human papillomavirus infection requires cell surface heparan sulfate. J Virol, 2001. **75**(3): pp. 1565-1570.

[33] DiMaio, D. and J.B. Liao, Human papillomaviruses and cervical cancer. Adv Virus Res, 2006. **66**: pp. 125-59.

[34] Burd, E.M., Human papillomavirus and cervical cancer. Clin Microbiol Rev, 2003. **16**(1): pp. 1-17.

[35] Chakrabarti, O. and S. Krishna, Molecular interactions of 'high risk' human papillomaviruses E6 and E7 oncoproteins: implications for tumour progression. J Biosci, 2003. **28**(3): pp. 337-48.

[36] Nuovo, G.J., et al., Strong inverse correlation between microRNA-125b and human papillomavirus DNA in productive infection. Diagn Mol Pathol, 2010. **19**(3): pp. 135-43.

[37] Zhang, B., D.F. Spandau, and A. Roman, E5 protein of human papillomavirus type 16 protects human foreskin keratinocytes from UV B-irradiation-induced apoptosis. J Virol, 2002. **76**(1): pp. 220-231.

[38] Mantovani, F. and L. Banks, The human papillomavirus E6 protein and its contribution to malignant progression. Oncogene, 2001. **20**(54): pp. 7874-87.

[39] Hawley-Nelson, P., et al., HPV16 E6 and E7 proteins cooperate to immortalize human foreskin keratinocytes. EMBO J, 1989. **8**(12): pp. 3905-10.

[40] Ishiji, T., Molecular mechanism of carcinogenesis by human papillomavirus-16. J Dermatol, 2000. **27**(2): pp. 73-86.

[41] zur Hausen, H., Papillomavirus infections—a major cause of human cancers. Biochim Biophys Acta, 1996. **1288**(2): pp. F55-78.

[42] Durst, M., et al., A papillomavirus DNA from a cervical carcinoma and its prevalence in cancer biopsy samples from different geographic regions. Proc Natl Acad Sci U S A, 1983. **80**(12): pp. 3812-5.

[43] Hanahan, D. and R.A. Weinberg, Hallmarks of cancer: the next generation. Cell, 2011. **144**(5): pp. 646-74.

[44] Calin, G.A. and C.M. Croce, MicroRNA signatures in human cancers. Nat Rev Cancer, 2006. **6**(11): pp. 857-66.

[45] Lee, J.W., et al., Altered MicroRNA expression in cervical carcinomas. Clin Cancer Res, 2008. **14**(9): pp. 2535-42.

[46] Wang, X., et al., Aberrant expression of oncogenic and tumor-suppressive microRNAs in cervical cancer is required for cancer cell growth. PLoS One, 2008. **3**(7): pp. e2557.

[47] Lui, W.O., et al., Patterns of known and novel small RNAs in human cervical cancer. Cancer Res, 2007. **67**(13): pp. 6031-43.

[48] Yamamoto, N., et al., Tumor suppressive microRNA-218 inhibits cancer cell migration and invasion by targeting focal adhesion pathways in cervical squamous cell carcinoma. Int J Oncol, 2013. **42**(5): pp. 1523-32.

[49] Rao, Q., et al., Aberrant microRNA expression in human cervical carcinomas. Med Oncol, 2012. **29**(2): pp. 1242-8.

[50] Li, J., Z. Ping, and H. Ning, MiR-218 impairs tumor growth and increases chemo-sensitivity to cisplatin in cervical cancer. Int J Mol Sci, 2012. **13**(12): pp. 16053-64.

[51] Kogo, R., et al., The microRNA-218~Survivin axis regulates migration, invasion, and lymph node metastasis in cervical cancer. Oncotarget, 2015. **6**(2): pp. 1090-100.

[52] Kozomara, A. and S. Griffiths-Jones, miRBase: annotating high confidence microRNAs using deep sequencing data. Nucleic Acids Res, 2014. **42**(Database issue): pp. D68-73.

[53] Hartmann, J.T. and H.P. Lipp, Toxicity of platinum compounds. Expert Opin Pharmacother, 2003. **4**(6): pp. 889-901.

[54] Eifel, P.J., Chemoradiotherapy in the treatment of cervical cancer. Semin Radiat Oncol, 2006. **16**(3): pp. 177-85.

[55] Sun, H., et al., Potential molecular mechanisms for improved prognosis and outcome with neoadjuvant chemotherapy prior to laparoscopical radical hysterectomy for patients with cervical cancer. Cell Physiol Biochem, 2013. **32**(5): pp. 1528-40.

[56] Smela, M.E., et al., The aflatoxin B(1) formamidopyrimidine adduct plays a major role in causing the types of mutations observed in human hepatocellular carcinoma. Proc Natl Acad Sci U S A, 2002. **99**(10): pp. 6655-60.

[57] Cadet, J., et al., Oxidatively generated complex DNA damage: tandem and clustered lesions. Cancer Lett, 2012. **327**(1-2): pp. 5-15.

[58] Roos, W.P. and B. Kaina, DNA damage-induced cell death: from specific DNA lesions to the DNA damage response and apoptosis. Cancer Lett, 2013. **332**(2): pp. 237-48.

[59] Adams, M., et al., Chemotherapy for ovarian cancer—a consensus statement on standard practice. Br J Cancer, 1998. **78**(11): p. 1404-6.

[60] De Pree, N. and J. Wils, Long-term survival of patients with advanced ovarian carcinoma treated with cisplatin-based chemotherapy regimens. Anticancer Res, 1989. **9**(6): pp. 1869-71.

[61] Bircher, J., The many effects of lactulose: a rational approach to its therapeutic use. Drugs, 1972. **4**(1): pp. 1-3.

[62] Siddik, Z.H., Cisplatin: mode of cytotoxic action and molecular basis of resistance. Oncogene, 2003. **22**(47): pp. 7265-79.

[63] Kelland, L.R., Preclinical perspectives on platinum resistance. Drugs, 2000. **59 Suppl 4**: pp. 1-8; discussion 37-8.

[64] Cardinaal, R.M., et al., Dose-dependent effect of 8-day cisplatin administration upon the morphology of the albino guinea pig cochlea. Hear Res, 2000. **144**(1-2): pp. 135-46.

[65] Ciarimboli, G., et al., Cisplatin nephrotoxicity is critically mediated via the human organic cation transporter 2. Am J Pathol, 2005. **167**(6): pp. 1477-84.

[66] Pabla, N., et al., The copper transporter Ctr1 contributes to cisplatin uptake by renal tubular cells during cisplatin nephrotoxicity. Am J Physiol Renal Physiol, 2009. **296**(3): pp. F505-11.

[67] Rosenberg, B., Fundamental studies with cisplatin. Cancer, 1985. **55**(10): pp. 2303–l6.

[68] Wang, D. and S.J. Lippard, Cellular processing of platinum anticancer drugs. Nat Rev Drug Discov, 2005. **4**(4): pp. 307-20.

[69] Fichtinger-Schepman, A.M., et al., Adducts of the antitumor drug cis-diamminedichloro platinum(II) with DNA: formation, identification, and quantitation. Biochemistry, 1985. **24**(3): pp. 707-13.

[70] Lippard, S.J. and J.D. Hoeschele, Binding of cis- and trans-dichlorodiammineplatinum(II) to the nucleosome core. Proc Natl Acad Sci U S A, 1979. **76**(12): pp. 6091-5.

[71] Corda, Y., et al., RNA polymerases react differently at d(ApG) and d(GpG) adducts in DNA modified by cis-diamminedichloroplatinum(II). Biochemistry, 1992. **31**(7): pp. 1904-8.

[72] Murray, V., et al., The use of Taq DNA polymerase to determine the sequence specificity of DNA damage caused by cis-diamminedichloroplatinum(II), acridine-tethered platinum(II) diammine complexes or two analogues. J Biol Chem, 1992. **267**(26): pp. 18805-9.

[73] Murray, V., J. Whittaker, and W.D. McFadyen, DNA sequence selectivity of cisplatin analogues in intact human cells. Chem Biol Interact, 1998. **110**(1-2): pp. 27-37.

[74] Roberts, J.J. and A.J. Thomson, The mechanism of action of antitumor platinum compounds. Prog Nucleic Acid Res Mol Biol, 1979. **22**: pp. 71-133.

[75] Rebbaa, A., et al., The role of histone acetylation versus DNA damage in drug-induced senescence and apoptosis. Cell Death Differ, 2006. **13**(11): pp. 1960-7.

[76] Van Waes, C., Nuclear factor-kappaB in development, prevention, and therapy of cancer. Clin Cancer Res, 2007. **13**(4): pp. 1076-82.

[77] Notarbartolo, M., et al., Antitumor effects of curcumin, alone or in combination with cisplatin or doxorubicin, on human hepatic cancer cells. Analysis of their possible relationship to changes in NF-kB activation levels and in IAP gene expression. Cancer Lett, 2005. **224**(1): pp. 53-65.

[78] Chirnomas, D., et al., Chemosensitization to cisplatin by inhibitors of the Fanconi anemia/BRCA pathway. Mol Cancer Ther, 2006. **5**(4): pp. 952-61.

[79] Vorasubin, N., et al., Glossopharyngeal schwannomas: a 100 year review. Laryngoscope, 2009. **119**(1): pp. 26-35.

[80] Masuda, Y. and K. Kamiya, Molecular nature of radiation injury and DNA repair disorders associated with radiosensitivity. Int J Hematol, 2012. **95**(3): pp. 239-45.

[81] Redon, C.E., et al., Histone gammaH2AX and poly(ADP-ribose) as clinical pharmacodynamic biomarkers. Clin Cancer Res, 2010. **16**(18): pp. 4532-42.

[82] Aparicio, T., R. Baer, and J. Gautier, DNA double-strand break repair pathway choice and cancer. DNA Repair (Amst), 2014. **19**: pp. 169-75.

[83] Deckbar, D., P.A. Jeggo, and M. Lobrich, Understanding the limitations of radiation-induced cell cycle checkpoints. Crit Rev Biochem Mol Biol, 2011. **46**(4): pp. 271-83.

[84] Guo, G.S., et al., DNA repair and synthetic lethality. Int J Oral Sci, 2011. **3**(4): pp. 176-9.

[85] Wang, G., et al., Risk factor for clear cell renal cell carcinoma in Chinese population: a case-control study. Cancer Epidemiol, 2012. **36**(2): pp. 177-82.

[86] Roos, W.P., A.D. Thomas, and B. Kaina, DNA damage and the balance between survival and death in cancer biology. Nat Rev Cancer, 2016. **16**(1): pp. 20-33.

[87] Langerak, P. and P. Russell, Regulatory networks integrating cell cycle control with DNA damage checkpoints and double-strand break repair. Philos Trans R Soc Lond B Biol Sci, 2011. **366**(1584): pp. 3562-71.

[88] Rogakou, E.P., et al., DNA double-stranded breaks induce histone H2AX phosphorylation on serine 139. J Biol Chem, 1998. **273**(10): pp. 5858-68.

[89] Phuah, N.H., et al., Alterations of microRNA expression patterns in human cervical carcinoma cells (Ca Ski) toward 1'S-1'-acetoxychavicol acetate and cisplatin. Reprod Sci, 2013. **20**(5): pp. 567-78.

[90] Cha, H.J., et al., Identification of ionizing radiation-responsive microRNAs in the IM9 human B lymphoblastic cell line. Int J Oncol, 2009. **34**(6): pp. 1661-8.

[91] Faraonio, R., et al., A set of miRNAs participates in the cellular senescence program in human diploid fibroblasts. Cell Death Differ, 2012. **19**(4): pp. 713-21.

[92] Galluzzi, L., et al., miR-181a and miR-630 regulate cisplatin-induced cancer cell death. Cancer Res, 2010. **70**(5): pp. 1793-803.

[93] Josson, S., et al., Radiation modulation of microRNA in prostate cancer cell lines. Prostate, 2008. **68**(15): pp. 1599-606.

[94] Pothof, J., et al., MicroRNA-mediated gene silencing modulates the UV-induced DNA-damage response. EMBO J, 2009. **28**(14): pp. 2090-9.

[95] He, L., et al., A microRNA component of the p53 tumour suppressor network. Nature, 2007. **447**(7148): pp. 1130-4.

[96] Niu, J., et al., DNA damage induces NF-kappaB-dependent microRNA-21 up-regulation and promotes breast cancer cell invasion. J Biol Chem, 2012. **287**(26): pp. 21783-95.

[97] Aguda, B.D., et al., MicroRNA regulation of a cancer network: consequences of the feedback loops involving miR-17-92, E2F, and Myc. Proc Natl Acad Sci U S A, 2008. **105**(50): pp. 19678-83.

[98] Fukuda, T., et al., DEAD-box RNA helicase subunits of the Drosha complex are required for processing of rRNA and a subset of microRNAs. Nat Cell Biol, 2007. **9**(5): pp. 604-11.

[99] Gregory, R.I., et al., The Microprocessor complex mediates the genesis of microRNAs. Nature, 2004. **432**(7014): pp. 235-40.

[100] Boominathan, L., The guardians of the genome (p53, TA-p73, and TA-p63) are regulators of tumor suppressor miRNAs network. Cancer Metastasis Rev, 2010. **29**(4): pp. 613-39.

[101] Trabucchi, M., et al., The RNA-binding protein KSRP promotes the biogenesis of a subset of microRNAs. Nature, 2009. **459**(7249): pp. 1010-4.

[102] Francia, S., et al., Site-specific DICER and DROSHA RNA products control the DNA-damage response. Nature, 2012. **488**(7410): pp. 231-5.

[103] Wei, W., et al., A role for small RNAs in DNA double-strand break repair. Cell, 2012. **149**(1): pp. 101-12.

[104] Liu, Y. and X. Lu, Non-coding RNAs in DNA damage response. Am J Cancer Res, 2012. **2**(6): pp. 658-75.

[105] Li, Z., et al., MiR-27a modulates MDR1/P-glycoprotein expression by targeting HIPK2 in human ovarian cancer cells. Gynecol Oncol, 2010. **119**(1): pp. 125-30.

[106] Kovalchuk, O., et al., Involvement of microRNA-451 in resistance of the MCF-7 breast cancer cells to chemotherapeutic drug doxorubicin. Mol Cancer Ther, 2008. **7**(7): pp. 2152-9.

[107] Feng, D.D., et al., Down-regulated miR-331-5p and miR-27a are associated with chemotherapy resistance and relapse in leukaemia. J Cell Mol Med, 2011. **15**(10): pp. 2164-75.

[108] Chen, Z., et al., MiR-27a modulates the MDR1/P-glycoprotein expression by inhibiting FZD7/beta-catenin pathway in hepatocellular carcinoma cells. Cell Signal, 2013. **25**(12): pp. 2693-701.

[109] Zhao, X., et al., miR-138 might reverse multidrug resistance of leukemia cells. Leuk Res, 2010. **34**(8): pp. 1078-82.

[110] Bao, L., et al., Increased expression of P-glycoprotein and doxorubicin chemoresistance of metastatic breast cancer is regulated by miR-298. Am J Pathol, 2012. **180**(6): pp. 2490-503.

[111] Xu, Y., et al., Changes in the expression of miR-381 and miR-495 are inversely associated with the expression of the MDR1 gene and development of multi-drug resistance. PLoS One, 2013. **8**(11): p. e82062.

[112] Yu, Y., et al., microRNA 30A promotes autophagy in response to cancer therapy. Autophagy, 2012. **8**(5): pp. 853-5.

[113] Zhang, Y., et al., Regulation of autophagy by miR-30d impacts sensitivity of anaplastic thyroid carcinoma to cisplatin. Biochem Pharmacol, 2014. **87**(4): pp. 562-70.

[114] Sumbul, A.T., et al., miR-204-5p expression in colorectal cancer: an autophagy-associated gene. Tumour Biol, 2014. **35**(12): pp. 12713-9.

[115] Chatterjee, A., D. Chattopadhyay, and G. Chakrabarti, MiR-16 targets Bcl-2 in paclitaxel-resistant lung cancer cells and overexpression of miR-16 along with miR-17 causes unprecedented sensitivity by simultaneously modulating autophagy and apoptosis. Cell Signal, 2015. **27**(2): pp. 189-203.

[116] Huang, N., et al., MiR-15a and miR-16 induce autophagy and enhance chemosensitivity of Camptothecin. Cancer Biol Ther, 2015. **16**(6): pp. 941-8.

[117] Zhao, J., et al., MiR-181a suppresses autophagy and sensitizes gastric cancer cells to cisplatin. Gene, 2016. **576**(2 Pt 2): pp. 828-33.

[118] Tsuchiya, Y., et al., MicroRNA regulates the expression of human cytochrome P450 1B1. Cancer Res, 2006. **66**(18): pp. 9090-8.

[119] Martinez, V.G., et al., CYP1B1 expression is induced by docetaxel: effect on cell viability and drug resistance. Br J Cancer, 2008. **98**(3): pp. 564-70.

[120] Mu, W., et al., miR-27b synergizes with anticancer drugs via p53 activation and CYP1B1 suppression. Cell Res, 2015. **25**(4): pp. 477-95.

[121] Choi, Y.M., et al., CYP1A1 is a target of miR-892a-mediated post-transcriptional repression. Int J Oncol, 2012. **41**(1): pp. 331-6.

[122] Boni, V., et al., miR-192/miR-215 influence 5-fluorouracil resistance through cell cycle-mediated mechanisms complementary to its post-transcriptional thymidilate synthase regulation. Mol Cancer Ther, 2010. **9**(8): pp. 2265-75.

[123] Maftouh, M., et al., miR-211 modulates gemcitabine activity through downregulation of ribonucleotide reductase and inhibits the invasive behavior of pancreatic cancer cells. Nucleosides Nucleotides Nucleic Acids, 2014. **33**(4-6): pp. 384-93.

[124] Mansour, W.Y., et al., Aberrant overexpression of miR-421 downregulates ATM and leads to a pronounced DSB repair defect and clinical hypersensitivity in SKX squamous cell carcinoma. Radiother Oncol, 2013. **106**(1): pp. 147-54.

[125] Yamakuchi, M. and C.J. Lowenstein, MiR-34, SIRT1 and p53: the feedback loop. Cell Cycle, 2009. **8**(5): pp. 712-5.

[126] Ivanovska, I., et al., MicroRNAs in the miR-106b family regulate p21/CDKN1A and promote cell cycle progression. Mol Cell Biol, 2008. **28**(7): pp. 2167-74.

[127] Wu, S., et al., Multiple microRNAs modulate p21Cip1/Waf1 expression by directly targeting its 3′ untranslated region. Oncogene, 2010. **29**(15): pp. 2302-8.

[128] Wang, X., et al., miR-424 acts as a tumor radiosensitizer by targeting aprataxin in cervical cancer. Oncotarget, 2016. **7**(47): pp. 77508-77515.

[129] Song, L., et al., miR-375 Modulates Radiosensitivity of HR-HPV-Positive Cervical Cancer Cells by Targeting UBE3A through the p53 Pathway. Med Sci Monit, 2015. **21**: pp. 2210-7.

[130] Shen, Y., et al., miR-375 is upregulated in acquired paclitaxel resistance in cervical cancer. Br J Cancer, 2013. **109**(1): pp. 92-9.

[131] Chen, Y., et al., MicroRNA-181a enhances the chemoresistance of human cervical squamous cell carcinoma to cisplatin by targeting PRKCD. Exp Cell Res, 2014. **320**(1): pp. 12-20.

[132] Li, J., et al., MicroRNA-218 increases cellular sensitivity to Rapamycin via targeting Rictor in cervical cancer. APMIS, 2015. **123**(7): pp. 562-70.

[133] Liu, J., et al., Knock-down of NDRG2 sensitizes cervical cancer Hela cells to cisplatin through suppressing Bcl-2 expression. BMC Cancer, 2012. **12**: pp. 370.

[134] Yu, Q., et al., miR-126 Suppresses the proliferation of cervical cancer cells and alters cell sensitivity to the chemotherapeutic drug bleomycin. Asian Pac J Cancer Prev, 2014. **14**(11): pp. 6569-72.

[135] Fan, Z., et al., MiR-125a promotes paclitaxel sensitivity in cervical cancer through altering STAT3 expression. Oncogenesis, 2016. **5**: pp. e197.

[136] Shi, M., et al., Glucocorticoid regulation of a novel HPV-E6-p53-miR-145 pathway modulates invasion and therapy resistance of cervical cancer cells. J Pathol, 2012. **228**(2): pp. 148-57.

[137] Pedroza-Torres, A., et al., A microRNA expression signature for clinical response in locally advanced cervical cancer. Gynecol Oncol, 2016. **142**(3): pp. 557-65.

[138] Hu, X., et al., A microRNA expression signature for cervical cancer prognosis. Cancer Res, 2010. **70**(4): pp. 1441-8.

[139] Zhang, B., et al., A specific miRNA signature promotes radioresistance of human cervical cancer cells. Cancer Cell Int, 2013. **13**(1): pp. 118.

[140] How, C., et al., Developing a prognostic micro-RNA signature for human cervical carcinoma. PLoS One, 2015. **10**(4): pp. e0123946.

[141] Oyagbemi, A.A., A.B. Saba, and A.O. Ibraheem, Curcumin: from food spice to cancer prevention. Asian Pac J Cancer Prev, 2009. **10**(6): pp. 963-7.

[142] Dai, X.Z., et al., Potential therapeutic efficacy of curcumin in liver cancer. Asian Pac J Cancer Prev, 2013. **14**(6): pp. 3855-9.

[143] Anuchapreeda, S., et al., Modulation of P-glycoprotein expression and function by curcumin in multidrug-resistant human KB cells. Biochem Pharmacol, 2002. **64**(4): pp. 573-82.

[144] Anand, P., et al., Bioavailability of curcumin: problems and promises. Mol Pharm, 2007. **4**(6): pp. 807-18.

[145] Roy, M. and S. Mukherjee, Reversal of resistance towards cisplatin by curcumin in cervical cancer cells. Asian Pac J Cancer Prev, 2014. **15**(3): pp. 1403-10.

[146] Promraksa, B., et al., Anticancer Potential of Cratoxylum formosum Subsp. Pruniflorum (Kurz.) Gogel Extracts Against Cervical Cancer Cell Lines. Asian Pac J Cancer Prev, 2015. **16**(14): pp. 6117-21.

[147] Maisuthisakul, P., R. Pongsawatmanit, and M.H. Gordon, Antioxidant properties of Teaw (Cratoxylum formosum Dyer) extract in soybean oil and emulsions. J Agric Food Chem, 2006. **54**(7): pp. 2719-25.

[148] Lirdprapamongkol, K., et al., Chrysin overcomes TRAIL resistance of cancer cells through Mcl-1 downregulation by inhibiting STAT3 phosphorylation. Int J Oncol, 2013. **43**(1): pp. 329-37.

[149] Spoerlein-Guettler, C., et al., Ferrocene and (arene)ruthenium(II) complexes of the natural anticancer naphthoquinone plumbagin with enhanced efficacy against resistant cancer cells and a genuine mode of action. J Inorg Biochem, 2014. **138**: pp. 64-72.

[150] Wei, D.D., J.S. Wang, and L.Y. Kong, Reversal effects of components from the fruits of Illicium simonsii on human Adriamycin-resistant MCF-7 and 5-fluorouracil-resistant Bel7402 cells. Phytother Res, 2012. **26**(4): pp. 562-7.

[151] Staerk, D., et al., In vitro cytotoxic activity of phenanthroindolizidine alkaloids from Cynanchum vincetoxicum and Tylophora tanakae against drug-sensitive and multi-drug-resistant cancer cells. J Nat Prod, 2002. **65**(9): pp. 1299-302.

Section 4

Precancer/cancer Treatment

Chapter 7

The Role of miRNAs in Diagnosis, Prognosis and Treatment Prediction in Cervical Cancer

Ovidiu Balacescu, Loredana Balacescu,
Oana Baldasici, Oana Tudoran and
Patriciu Achimas-Cadariu

Additional information is available at the end of the chapter

http://dx.doi.org/10.5772/68011

Abstract

Cervical cancer represents one of the major problems of health women worldwide, especially in the developing countries. If discovered in its earliest stages, cervical cancer is successfully treatable; however, due to lack of proper implementation of screening programs, the majority of cervical cancer patients are diagnosed in advanced stages, which dramatically influence their outcome. Almost a half of these patients will suffer recurrence or metastasis in the following 2 years after therapy. If there are no immediate prospects in terms of developing new or more effective therapies, identifying new tools for early diagnosis, prognosis and treatment prediction remains a big challenge for cervical cancer. miRNAs have been validated to be key players in cell physiology, alterations in miRNA expression being associated with cancer progression and response to therapy. Cervical cancer studies have showed that alterations of miRNA expression can be identified in tumor tissues, exfoliated cervical cells and patients serum and that their transcription pattern is regulated by the present HPV genotype. Furthermore, miRNAs have been associated with patients response to therapy, therefore suggesting their potential to be used as biomarkers for cervical cancer diagnosis, prognosis and treatment response.

Keywords: cervical cancer, miRNA, HPV, Diagnosis, Prognosis, treatment response

1. Introduction

With an incidence of over a half million new cases every year, cervical cancer still represents a major health problem for women worldwide. The last collected data from 2012 show that the incidence is not proportionally distributed, 84% of new cases (444,500 out of 527,600)

being recorded in developing countries and only 16% new cases in developed ones [1]. Consequently, the mortality rate is pretty similar, with 86.63% deaths (230,200 of 265,700) recorded in developing areas, compared with 13.47% deaths registered in developed ones.

This burden is related to the dis-proportional implementation of screening programs (Pap smear and HPV tests), which allow the early detection of cervical precancerous and cancerous lesions that can be successfully treated surgically. Previous data revealed that cervical cancer control programs based on Pap test reduce the risk of cervical cancer with 25–36% [2]. To maximize the screening effect, World Human Organization (WHO) recommended Pap test for women 30 years or older, considered at high risk for developing cervical cancer. Moreover, testing and following the patients with persistent high-risk HPV infections could identify the early stages of cervical cancer.

Unfortunately, due to lack of proper implementation of screening programs in developing areas, the majority of cervical cancer patients are diagnosed in locally advanced stages (IIB–IIIB). Depending on the stage of the disease, the treatment includes radiotherapy concomitant with adjuvant or neoadjuvant chemotherapy, associated or not with surgery [3]. Nevertheless, the advanced stages will dramatically influence their response to the therapy, and almost a half of these patients will suffer recurrence or metastasis in the following 2 years after treatment.

In cervical cancer, as in the other cancers, the identification of new competitive drugs and new accurate biomarkers for diagnosis and prognosis is challenging. If there are no immediate prospects regarding developing new or more effective drug-based therapies, identifying new tools for early diagnosis, prognosis or treatment predictions, has become a necessity.

The genomics revolution has uncovered new molecular data that advanced the characterization and the understanding of the complex regulatory signaling networks that drive cancer growth and development. Molecular findings related to both coding and non-coding transcriptome were investigated in order to identify new cancer biomarkers, including in cervical cancer. Of these, non-coding RNAs related to cell functionality, such as micro RNA (miRNA), have became important pieces of puzzle to characterize cervical cancer phenotype or to investigate their involvement in prognosis and treatment response.

The subsequent chapter will present the existent data regarding the involvement of miRNAs in cervical carcinogenesis, including their synthesis, stability and specificity, as well as the role of HPVs infection in modulating host's miRNAs expression. Furthermore, we will discuss the latest updates on the miRNAs clinical applications as additional valuable markers for diagnosis, prognosis and treatment prediction in cervical cancer.

2. Micro-RNAs

MiRNAs represent a class of non-coding RNAs, evolutionary conserved between species, which negatively regulate gene expression at both transcriptional and post-transcriptional levels, during normal and pathological conditions [4, 5]. Functional studies indicate that up to 60% of protein-coding genes (PCGs) are regulated by miRNAs, which "gained" them the name of "master modulators" of the human genome [6, 7]. An interesting aspect of miRNAs is that each miRNA can target up to 200 mRNAs on average or different miRNAs can target the same mRNA [8]. In physiological conditions, miRNAs play important roles in the modulation of many cellular processes and mechanisms such as angiogenesis, cell cycle regulation, differentiation, apoptosis, DNA repair or stress response. Subsequently, when alterations occur in their expression, miRNAs become key regulators of many diseases, including cancer. Several genetic and epigenetic events induce changes in miRNAs expression, including DNA amplifications or deletions that lead to gain or loss of miRNAs loci regions. Moreover, DNA mutations or SNPs (single nucleotide polymorphisms) inside of miRNAs coding genes could modify the miRNAs specificity by changing their structure [9]. Epigenetic modifications are related to hypermethylation of CpG islands of the transcriptional factors and promoters of miRNA-coding genes resulting in silencing of these genes, leading to miRNAs expression alteration [10]. Croce's group demonstrated for the first time an association of miRNAs with cancer, identifying deletion and down-regulation of two miRNAs (miR-15 and miR-16) in 13q14 LOH (Loss of Heterozygosity) of chronic lymphocytic leukemia [11]. The same group demonstrated that the majority of miRNAs genes are located in cancer-associated genomic regions, considered genomic fragile sites [12]. Taking advantage of high-throughput microarray technology, Calin et al. [13] demonstrated that genome-wide miRNA profiling represents a reliable tool to characterize and investigate tumor phenotypes, deepening the understanding of the molecular mechanisms of cancer. Since 1993, when the first miRNAs were discovered, extensive research and tremendous efforts were put into identifying and characterizing new miRNAs. Due to the identification of growing numbers of miRNAs, a miRNA database was assembled, the miRBase Release 2.0 including 506 miRNA sequences from six organisms became firstly available in 2004 via web interface [14]. Currently, 26,654 entries from 223 species, including 2588 mature human miRNAs, have been deposited in the newest data from miRBase Release 21 (http://www.mirbase.org/).

2.1. Biogenesis of miRNA

It is estimated that only a small fraction (less than 2%) of the human genome is represented by coding DNA (exons from PCGs), while the rest of 98% include sequences of non-coding DNA such as introns, non-coding RNAs, regulatory DNA sequences, and other DNA sequences with unknown functions [15]. Non-coding DNAs play important roles in controlling all steps of gene expression, when PCGs are transcribed into mRNAs and translated into proteins. The investigation of functions of non-coding DNAs during the ENCODE (Encyclopedia of DNA Elements) project revealed new data related to how genetic information is converted into living cells and also the fact that almost 80% of human genome is activate in cell physiology [16]. Part of non-coding RNAs, miRNAs represent the most studied components being widely accepted that they are major players in cell cycle dynamics, regardless of the physiological or pathological status.

Generally, almost all regions of the genome may encode miRNA. As much as 40% of miRNAs are located in intragenic regions, within the introns or even in the exons of the PCGs. The majority of the miRNAs (50%) are encoded by both intronic (40%) and exonic (10%) regions of non-protein coding genes also known as non-protein coding RNAs (npcRNAs) (**Figure 1**) [17].

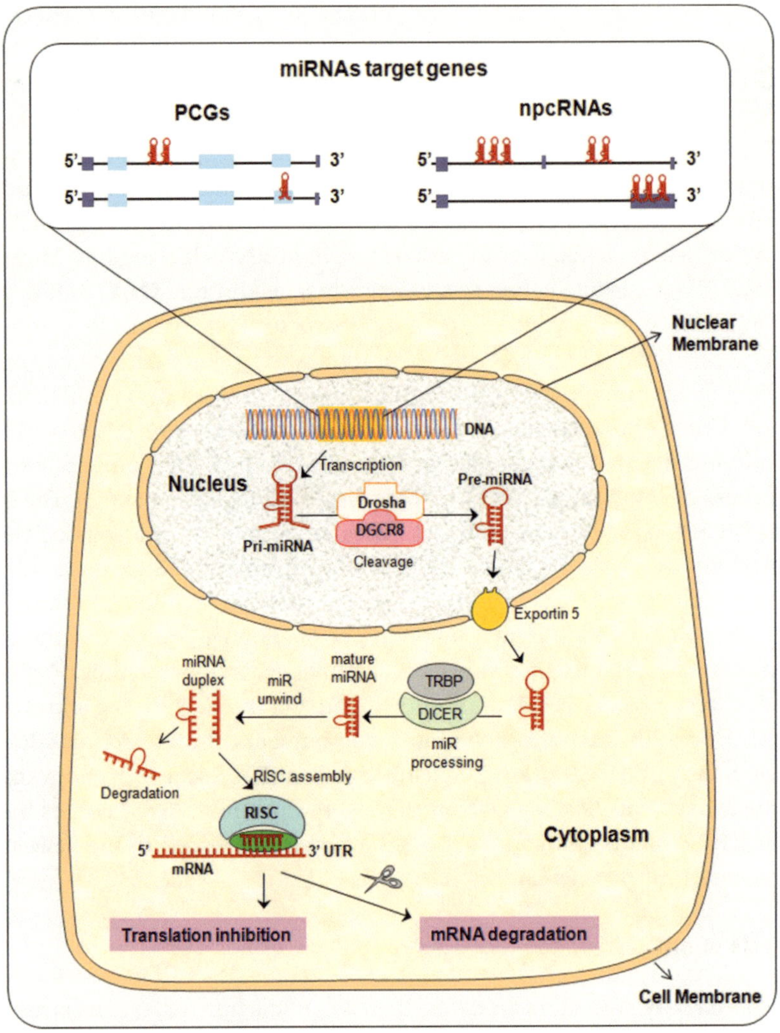

Figure 1. The biogenesis of miRNAs. MiRNAs are transcribed from intra- and intergenic regions of DNA, from both PCGs and npcRNAs. The long hairpins structures (pri-miRNA) transcribed from DNA are cleaved in pre-miRNAs smaller transcripts (~70 nucleotides long) by a microprocessor complex that includes Drosha and DGCR8 enzymes. After nuclear export through exportin 5, pre-miRNAs are processed to mature miRNAs. One miRNA strand is loaded in RNA-induced silencing complex (RISC) complex, while the other is degraded. RISC complex aligns by sequence complementarity to the target mRNA and negatively regulate their expression by degradation and/or translational repression.

The miRNAs transcription starts in the nucleus being mediated by RNA polymerase II [18], but there is also some evidence that miRNAs could be transcribed by RNA polymerase III when are associated with Alu family repetitive elements [19]. The first miRNA transcripts (pri-miRNAs) transcribed from DNA are long hairpin structures that include hundreds or thousands nucleotides. Upon recognition of a microprocessor complex, including RNA polymerase III Drosha and DGCR8 (DiGeorge syndrome critical region 8), pri-miRNAs are processed into one or more smaller hairpins of about 70 nucleotides long called precursor miRNAs (pre-miRNAs) [20]. Forward, pre-miRNAs are exported from nucleus to the cytoplasm by the nuclear export receptor exportin 5 [21]. After their export in cytoplasm, pre-miRNAs are processed by cytoplasmic RNA polymerase III Dicer to generate 21–23 nucleotides mature miRNA duplexes [22]. The miRNA strand with less stable paired 5′ end will be preferentially loaded into Argonaute 2 (AGO2) proteins that possess cleavage activity, while the other miRNA strand will be degraded [23]. The miRNA-loaded AGO2 protein will be incorporated into RNA-induced silencing complex (RISC) that will target by sequence complementarity to the 3′UTR of specific mRNA target, leading to mRNA degradation or translational repression.

2.2. MiRNAs in cancer

Non-coding RNAs, especially miRNAs, have changed the sense of the "central dogma of molecular biology." In accordance with central dogma of molecular biology, RNAs represent intermediary information in the genetic flow, by copying genetic information (transcription) from DNA and transform it (translation) to cellular effectors, the proteins:

$$\begin{gathered}\textbf{DNA} \rightarrow \text{transcription} \rightarrow \textbf{mRNA} \rightarrow \text{translation} \rightarrow \textbf{Proteins} \\ (\text{the central dogma of molecular biology})\end{gathered} \tag{1}$$

Following discovery and characterization of small non-coding RNA, such as miRNAs, siRNAs and piwi RNAs as well as long non-coding RNAs and ultraconserved elements (UCEs), the central dogma of molecular biology has became more complex [24]. Actually, the genetic information from DNA is transcribed in both coding RNAs (mRNAs) and non-coding RNAs (miRNAs, siRNAs, piwiRNAs, lncRNAs and ECEs). Furthermore, ncRNAs actively participate both in the regulation of protein synthesis by regulation of the DNA transcription and mRNA translation as well as by regulating their expression by complex cross-regulation [16] (**Figure 2**).

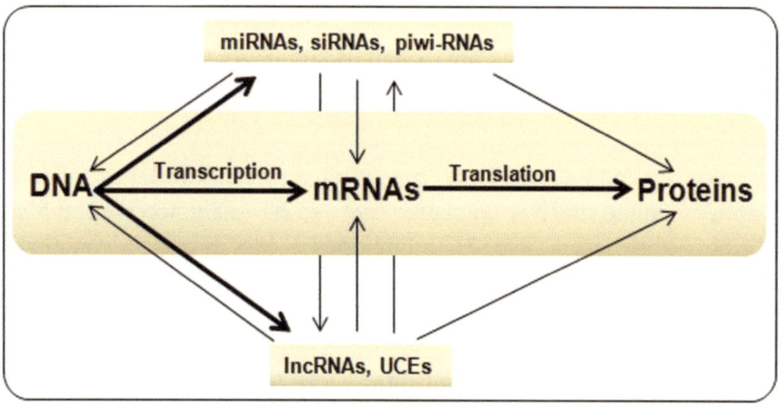

Figure 2. The new concept of the central dogma of molecular biology. The genetic information from DNA is transcribed (bold arrows) in both coding RNAs (mRNAs) and non-coding RNAs (miRNAs, siRNAs, piwiRNAs, lncRNAs and ECEs), while the mRNA translation in their specific proteins includes complex regulations (regular arrows) performed by all type of ncRNAs.

After their discovery, miRNAs have become a hot subject for many researchers worldwide, in the attempt to establish their role in cell functionality, especially in cancer. Croce's lab was the first that established that miRNAs alteration can be associated with cancer [11], showing that miR-15 and miR-16 were deleted or down-regulated in the majority of patients with chronic lymphocytic leukemia. Furthermore, they demonstrated that these miRNAs act as tumor suppressor genes, inducing apoptosis of leukemic tumor cells by negatively regulation of the expression of BCL2 oncogene (mRNA), which encodes a protein that blocks the apoptotic death [25]. The expression of both miR-15 and miR-16 was inversely correlated with Bcl2 expression, strengthening the hypothesis that miRNAs are post-transcriptional negative regulators their mRNA targets and can be successfully used to characterize malignant hematological tumors [13]. Immediately afterwards, miRNA profiling has quickly become an important tool to characterize tumor phenotype and identify specific miRNA biomarkers. MiRNAs were clearly related to cancer development by three landmark studies published in Nature. In one of these studies, Lu et al. [26] demonstrated that poorly differentiated tumors are successfully classified when miRNA profiling is used; moreover, miRNA profiling represents better classifiers than mRNA profiling. In the second landmark study, He et al. [27] demonstrated that miR-17-92 cluster has an oncogenic potential, and its expression can modulate carcinogenesis in B-cell lymphoma in synergy with c-myc transcriptor factor. Although the mechanism of the oncogenic effect has not been fully elucidated, the authors suggested a decrease of apoptosis in these cells. The mechanisms that underlie the synergy between c-myc and miR-17-19b overexpression in B-cell lymphomas were demonstrated 10 years later by Mihailovich et al. [28] based on a comprehensive analysis integrating proteomics, transcriptomics and miRNAs prediction analysis. The third landmark study performed by O'Donnell et al. [29] demonstrated that the activity of E2F1 transcriptional factor can be controlled by two clusters of miRNAs (mir-17 and mir-106a) whose expression is activated by c-myc oncogene. After miRNAs were definitively linked to cancer development, a worldwide research effort has been made to characterize and establish the miRNAs roles in cancer.

Collectively, all previous data showed that miRNAs represent key ubiquitous players involved in cancer development. MiRNAs regulate molecular pathways involved in all cancer hallmarks such as self-sufficiency in growth signals, indolence to antigrowth signals, evasion from apoptosis, limitless potential replicative, angiogenesis, invasion and metastasis, reprogramming energy metabolism and evading immune destruction [30].

The growing miRNA profiling data, target prediction and data validation led to the development of specialized online miRNA databases that can be easily accessed in a user-friendly manner. Until now, there are at least 14 online open-access databases containing extensive information about miRNAs [31]. Some of these databases (*SomammiR DB2.0*) are useful to search for miRNAs somatic mutations and to predict their functional analysis based on these mutations, to identify miRNAs alterations involved in protein regulation (CancerNet) or to review the annotation changes for each miRNAs entry (miRbase Tracker). Additional databases focus on miRNAs roles in particular types of cancer such as head and neck and oral carcinomas (HNOCDB), endometrial (miREC), renal (Renal Cancer cell database), pancreatic (Pancreatic Cancer Database), sarcoma (Sarcoma microRNA Expression Database) or breast cancers (OncomiRdbB). Certain miRNA databases such as canEvolve include recent information from next-generation sequencing (NGS) technology in different type of cancers, healthy people and other pathologies, while miRCancer stores data about miRNAs in cancers collected by data mining. Other miRNAs databases are focused on the role of miRNAs in diagnosis and overall survival (PROGmiR) and their presence in extracellular vesicles (miRandola) as well as their role in autophagy activation (AutomiRDB).

2.3. MiRNAs can function as oncogenes or tumor suppressor genes

It is well known that cancer is a disease characterized by abnormal cell grown caused by uncontrolled division of cells. Two main classes of genes such as proto-oncogenes (ex KRAS, MYC, Her-2/neu, EGFR) and tumor-suppressor (ex RB, TP53, PTEN) are involved in the regulation of cell cycle in normal conditions.

When cancer occurs, multiple genetic and epigenetic alterations disrupt the normal function of these two classes of genes leading to their abnormal expression and therefore, uncontrolled cell division [32]. Cancer cells appear when proto-oncogenes are converted in oncogenes by "gain of function," and tumor-suppressor genes are inactivated or deleted resulting in "loss of function." From a functional perspective, the oncogenes and tumor suppresser genes expression can be modulated by miRNAs toward mRNA degradation or translational repression. Many previous studies have shown that miRNAs play both oncogene (oncomiR) and tumor-suppressor (tumor-suppressor miRNAs, TS-miRNAs) roles. By their up-regulation, onco-miRNAs negatively modulate the expression of tumor suppressor genes, while the down-regulation of TS-miRNAs will result in the absence of regulation or increased expression of oncogenes. A selection of oncomiRs and tumor-suppressor miRNAs, their mRNA targets as well as the pathologies where they are involved are presented in **Table 1**.

OncomiR or/tumor suppressor miR (TS-miR)	MiRNAs/ expression	Validated mRNA targets/regulation	miRNAs Function	Pathologies associated with miRNAs alteration	Ref.
oncomiR	miR-21↑	BCL2↓ PTEN↓ PDCD4↓ BTG2↓ TPM1↓	Promote cell survival and proliferation by antiapoptotic effects	Overexpressed in a variety of human tumors including breast, melanoma, ovarian, head and neck, colon, prostate, lung, pancreas and cervix	[33–37]
oncomiR	miR-155↑	PTEN↓ BCL2↓ SOCS1↓ SOCS6↓ BLC6↓	Induces cell proliferation, differentiation and migration, as well as inhibits apoptosis	Up-regulated in different cancers such as, breast, liver, hematological malignancies and cervix	[37–40]
oncomiR	miR-221/222↑	PTEN↓ TIMP3↓ $p27^{Kip1}$↓ CDKN1C/p57↓ BBC3/PUMA↓	Promotes cell proliferation, regulate cell cycle phase distribution, and inhibits apoptosis	Overexpressed in glioblastomas, thyroid papillary carcinomas, breast cancer, glioma, hepatocellular carcinoma, and lung cancer	[41]

OncomiR or/tumor suppressor miR (TS-miR)	MiRNAs/ expression	Validated mRNA targets/regulation	miRNAs Function	Pathologies associated with miRNAs alteration	Ref.
oncomiR	Cluster miR-17-92↑	PTEN↓ TGFBR2↓ SMAD2↓ SMAD4↓ P21↓	Promote tumorignesis, cell cycle progression, cell proliferation and survival	Up-regulation in glioblastoma, lymphomas as well as thyroid, pancreas, colorectal, breast, lung, and stomach cancers	[44, 45]
TS-miR	miR-221/222↓	c-Kit↓	Inhibits of erythropoiesis	Loss in erythroblastic leukemia	[42]
TS-miR	Cluster miR-17-92↓	AIB1↑	Suppress proliferation	Down-regulation in breast cancer	[46]
TS-miR	miR-15a↓ miR16-1↓	BCL2↑	Induces apoptosis, inhibits carcinogenesis	Deleted (loss) in chronic lymphocytic leukemia, prostate, breast and cervical cancers	[11, 47, 48]
TS-miR	miR-34↓	CCDC↑ CDK4↑ CDK6↑ HMGB1 Wnt/β↑	Induces apoptosis and inhibits cell proliferation, invasion and metastasis	Down-regulated in laryngeal, liver, pancreatic, colorectal, breast and cervical cancers	[50–52]
TS-miR	miR-143↓	KRAS↑ MMP-13↑ CD44v3↑ COX2↑ ERK5↑	Suppress proliferation, tumor development and proliferation, invasion and metastasis and induces apoptosis	Down-regulated in prostate, bladder, colon, breast and cervical cancers	[53, 54]
TS-miR	miR-145↓	ERG↑ FLI-1↑ KRAS↑ MUC1↑ IRS-1↑ VEGF-A↑	Suppress cell growth tumor invasion, proliferation angiogenesis and promotes apoptosis	Down-regulated in prostate, colon, breast, ovarian and cervical cancer	[55–57]

Table 1. Selection of oncomiRs and tumor suppressor miRNAs (TS-miR), their mRNA targets, and the pathologies were they are involved.

MiR-21, one of the most oncogenic miRNAs, is frequently overexpressed in many tumor types [33] including cervical cancer cells [34]. MiR-21 can down-regulate multiple tumor suppressor genes such as phosphatase and tensin homolog (PTEN), B-cell lymphoma protein 2 (BCL2), programmed cell death 4 (PDCD4), BTG2 or tropomyosin 2 (TPM2), leading to cell survival, increased proliferation and decreased apoptosis [35, 36].

MiR-155 is another oncomiR highly expressed in tumors, which negatively regulated multiple tumor suppressor genes such as PTEN, suppressor of cytokine signaling 1(SOCS1), suppressor of cytokine signaling (SOCS6), and B-cell CLL/lymphoma 6 (BCL6) [37–39]. In cervical cancer, high expression of miR-155 is associated with poor prognosis [40].

Two highly homologous microRNAs, miR-221 and miR-222, are key miRNAs deregulated in many types of cancers, having a double role as oncogenes or tumor suppressors depending on the cellular context and tumor type. In the majority of tumors where mir221/222 were identified, these act as oncomiRs by promoting cell proliferation, regulating cell cycle phase distribution, and inhibiting apoptosis. Their validated targets include several tumor suppressor genes such as PTEN, BCL2 binding component 3 (BBC3/PUMA) and TIMP metallopeptidase inhibitor 3 (TIMP3) tumor suppressor genes [41]. Contrary, in erythroleukemic cells, mir-221/222 has been showed to act as tumor-suppressors, by down-regulating proto-oncogene receptor tyrosine kinase (c-Kit), leading to inhibition of erythropoiesis [42].

Similar with miR221/222, miR-17-92 cluster was validated for both oncogenic and tumor suppressive roles [43]. The oncogenic activity of miR-17-92 cluster is related to the negative modulation of PTEN tumor suppressor gene [44], and multiple components of TGFβ signaling pathway, including transcriptional modulators such as SMAD2/SMAD4 and CDKNIA (p21) which are involved in negative regulation of cell cycle progression [45]. The suppressor role of miR-17-92 cluster was proved by its miR-17-5p member that negatively regulates the nuclear receptor coactivator 3 (NCOA3/AIB1), leading to decreased proliferation of breast cancer cells [46].

While some miRNAs promote carcinogenesis by their up-regulation, several studies have shown that the majority of tumors present deletions of miRNAs tumor suppressor genes, due to the fact that they are located in or near fragile sites of cancer-associated genomic regions, genomics rearrangements (chromosomal and/or genes) [12]. For example, the first cluster of tumor suppressor miRNAs (mir-15a/miR-16-1) was related to deletion of 13q14.3 region in chronic lymphocytic leukemia. Calin et al. [11] demonstrated that the expression of BCL2 oncoprotein (anti-apoptotic regulator), target of mir-15a/miR-16-1, is inversely correlated with these miRNAs. The role of miR-15 and mir-16 tumor suppressor genes was also demonstrated in prostate and breast cancer cells [47, 48] as well as in cervical cancers [49].

A component of TP53 tumor suppressor network, mir-34a represents another tumor suppressor gene that regulates cell proliferation by targeting cyclin D1 (CCDC1), cyclin-dependent kinase 4 (CDK4) and cyclin-dependent kinase 6 (CDK6) proteins or Wnt/β-catenin signaling pathway in laryngeal [50], breast [51] colon and cervical cancers [52].

Down-regulation or loss of function of miRNA-143 was identified in multiple cancers including cervical cancer, being associated with carcinogenesis and tumor progression [53]. Some important targets of miR-143 include KRAS proto-oncogene conducting cancer development, matrix metallopeptidase 13 (MMP-13) with role in metastasis, cluster of differentiation 44v3 (CD44v3) involved in migration and invasion, cyclooxygenase 2 (COX2) supporting tumor metastasis by tumor proliferation, migration and epithelial-mesenchymal transition (EMT) [54].

Tumor suppressor miR-145 has important roles in the regulation of cell proliferation, and its loss or down-regulation has been associated with development and progression as well as invasion and metastasis of different type of malignancies such as breast, ovarian, colon, prostate and cervical cancer [55, 56]. The mir-145 targets include erythroblast transformation-specific (ETS) family of transcriptions factors (ERG),

KRAS, fms-related tyrosine kinase 1 (FLT1), mucin 1 (MUC1), vascular endothelial growth factor A (VEGFA) and insulin receptor substrate 1, involved in different pathways of tumor progression and metastasis [57].

3. High-risk HPV infection modulates miRNA expression in cervical cancer

Human Papillomaviruses (HPVs) represent the most important risk factor for developing cervical cancer. Papillomaviruses are small (50–60 nm) DNA viruses, counting over 200 members that include more than 150 HPVs [58]. Depending on their type of infection, HPVs are divided into two subgroups: cutaneous, which infects cutaneous skin producing benign papillomas (warts), and mucosal, infecting mucosal epithelial cells, which provoke epithelial dysplasia and invasive carcinoma. Currently, 12 HPVs that include 16, 18, 31, 33, 35, 39, 45, 51, 52, 56, 58, 59 subtypes are confirmed oncogenic and referred to as high-risk HPVs (HR-HPVs) [59]. The infection and minimum 2 years persistence with HR-HPVs is a prior condition of cervical cancers. As a result of the discovery that HR-HPVs are causative agents of cervical cancer, Harald zur Hausen was awarded the Nobel Prize in 2008. Data from epidemiological studies revealed that HPV 16 and 18 subtypes are associated with the majority of cervical cancers [60]. Moreover, previous data showed that HPV detection increases during transition from precancerous lesions to cervical cancers. If in CIN1 (cervical intraepithelial neoplasia) characterized by low-grade dysplasia, HPV is present in proportion of 50–70%, in middle dysplasia (CIN2), it increases to 85%, while in severe dysplasia (CIN3) and cervical cancer, the HPV presence raises to almost 100% [61]. This observation was further exploited to identify HPV-dependent-specific biomarkers for cervical cancer detection.

Because the HPV genomes do not possess their own enzymes necessary for viral replication, these viruses will use the enzymatic machinery of the host infected cells (basal layer of squamous epithelia) to sustain DNA viral replication. HPVs possess small genomes, of about 8 kb in size, including a well-conserved core set of genes involved in replication (E1 and E2) and packaging (L1 and L2). The remaining HPV genome includes genes (E4, E5, E6, and E7) that modify cellular environment, cell cycle regulation, immune evasion, and virus release. The detailed roles of the proteins encoded by these genes, involving host cells infection, evading the immune system and the modulation of carcinogenic pathways were recently presented [59]. Shortly, following infection, HPVs have the ability to insert their genetic material into host's cell genome, leading to expression and replication of viral DNA by the host cell. Expression of viral genes E1 and E2 leads to the production of oncoproteins E5, E6, E7. These oncoproteins act in a cooperative way to promote malignant transformation of the host cell by inhibiting p53 and pRB tumor suppressor proteins, altering the apoptosis and the cell-cycle control, activating telomerase and promoting the proliferation of infected cells.

Cellular changes due to HR-HPVs are also visible in microRNA regulation. Several studies reported aberrant miRNA expression profiles in HPV positive cervical cancer when compared to HPV-negative cervical cancers. In particular, E6 and E7, but also E5 HR-HPV oncoproteins, are capable of modulating the expression of different miRNAs in host infected cervical cancer cells (**Figure 3**).

http://dx.doi.org/10.5772/68011

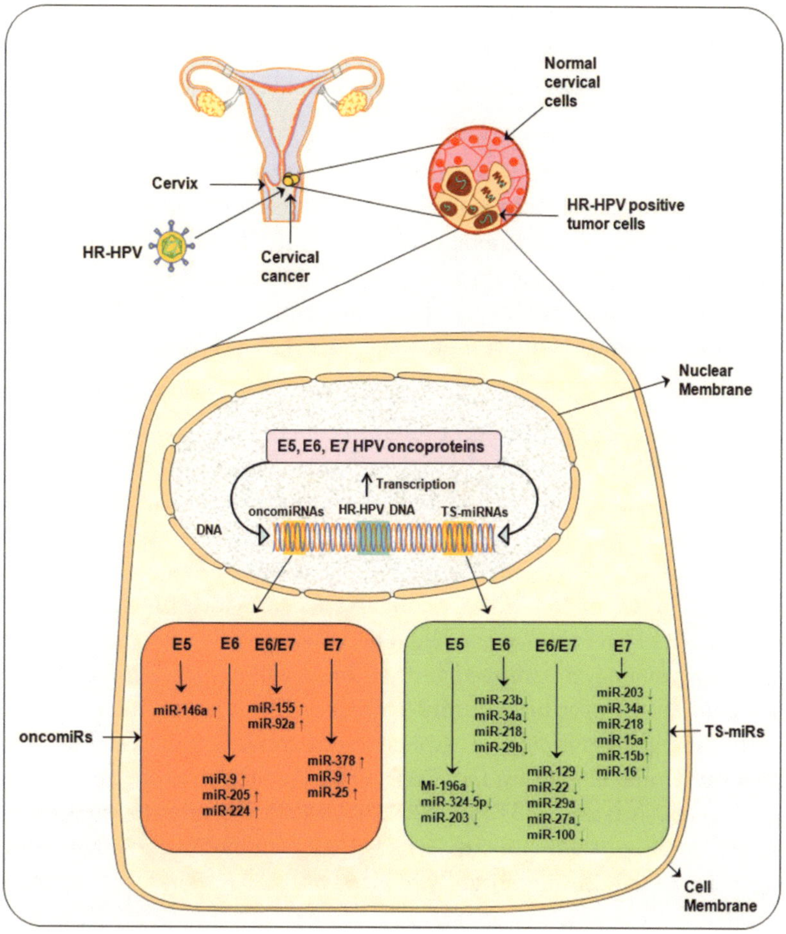

Figure 3. miRNAs modulated by HR-HPV E5, E6 and E7 oncoproteins in cervical cancer. After infecting the basal layer of squamous epithelia, HPV virus modifies the cellular environment, cell cycle regulation, cell proliferation and migration, immune evasion and altering the apoptosis by regulation of specific miRNAs. HPVs insert their genetic material into host's cell genome, leading to expression of specific sets of oncomiRs and blocking or modulating certain miRNAs, in a cooperative way that promote malignant transformation of the host cell.

In a study comprising 101 cervical cancer cases, Liu et al. [62] identified the E6 and E7 HPV transcripts in all the HPV-positive cases (86% of all cervical cancer samples). Four miRNAs, including miR-9, miR-205, miR-224 (up-regulated) and miR-29b (down-regulated), were correlated with HP-positive expression using HPV-negative cancers as controls. MiR-9 was selected for further investigations and validation as it was the most aberrantly expressed miRNA. Their results showed that miR-9 is mostly expressed by HPV16 infected cells, and it is mainly activated by E6, (up-regulated 45-fold as a result of E6 expression), but also due to E7 (5-fold up-regulation). Based on target prediction algorithms, RNA-seq data and RT-PCR experiments, they identified FASTL1 (involved in cellular proliferation) and ALCAM (involved in cell migration) as miR-9 targets in cervical cancer.

Au Yeung et al. [63] demonstrated in vitro that HPV16 E6 protein leads to the down-regulation of tumor suppressor miR-23b, through p53 degradation. The decreasing expression of miR-23b results in increasing expression of urokinase-type plasminogen activator (uPA) that leads to increased migration of cervical tumor cells. Moreover, the reduce expression of miR-23b was related to invasion and metastasis, being considered a prognostic factor of cervical carcinoma [64].

In a similar study, Raver-Shapira's group [65] demonstrated that HPV E6 oncoprotein can decrease the expression of miR-34a through p53 destabilization during viral infection. MiR-34a represents an important tumor suppressor miRNA, whose alteration leads to cell proliferation, by activating the genes involved in cell cycle regulation such as cyclins (E2 and D1), cyclin-dependent kinases (CDK4, CDK6), transcription factors (E2F1, E2F3, E2F5), and decreased apoptosis by up-regulation of antiapoptotic Bcl-2 [66, 67].

Another target of HPV16 E6 oncoprotein is miR-218. In vitro and in vivo studies demonstrated that miR-218 is down-regulated by E6 oncoprotein in both precancerous lesions and cervical cancers. In an in vivo study, Li's group [68] proposed to investigate whether there is a correlation between HPV16 infection and miR-218 down-regulation and to evaluate the relationship between miR-218 expression and CIN staging. Seventy-eight CIN cases were included in this study. Of all the cases, 66% presented infection with a single HPV type, 24% presented infection with multiple HPV subtypes, and 9% were HPV free. Quantitative RT-PCR measurements showed a down-regulation of miR-218 in CIN cases presenting HR-HPV infections compared to HPV-free CIN cases. MiR-218 expression levels dropped further down with CIN stage evolution, CIN3 cases presenting a significantly lower level of miR-218 than CIN1. One of the targets of miR-218 is LAMB3 with roles in cell migration and carcinogenesis of cervical cancer. Another study revealed that the expression of miR-218 can lead to EMT inhibition, migration and invasion by targeting pro-tumorigenic genes such as SFMBT1 and DCUN1D1 [69]. Recently, the expression of miR-218 in cervical cancer was associated with radiosensitivity via promoting radiation induced apoptosis, down-regulation of miR-218 significantly reduced the radiation-induced apoptosis [70].

If HR-HPV E6 oncoprotein mediates the miRNAs targets through p53 destabilization, the HR-HPV E7 oncoprotein modulates the miRNAs targets by increasing the transcription of E2F family of transcription factors through degradation of pRB from pRB-E2F complex, leading to releases and activation of transcription factor E2F [71]. In this regard, several miRNA targets of HR-HPV E7 oncoprotein such as miR-15a, miR-15b and miR-16 were identified as targets of E2F transcription factors [72, 73]. These miRNAs, considered tumor suppressor miRNAs (TS-miRNAs), were identified as overexpressed in cervical cancers. Interestingly, miR-15b was also suggested to play an important role in cervical carcinogenesis, regulating mechanisms such as angiogenesis, invasion and metastasis by targeting and down-regulating the RECK gene, which can negatively affect the transcription and activity of MMPs [74]. Another target of E7 oncoprotein is represented by miR-203, identified by Yi et al. [75]. Mir-203, by its p63 target, has an important role in regulating the proliferation of undifferentiated basal cells and repress "stemness" of epithelial cells.

To identify new targets of HR-HPV E6 and E7 oncoproteins, Wang et al. [76] established an in vitro study based on miR-array and miR-seq exploratory analysis, followed by data validation on human samples. They identified in cell culture a set of 13 statistically significant miRNAs (miR-16, miR-25, miR-92a, miR-83, miRr-106b, miR-210, miR-224, miR-378, miR-22, miR-24, miR-27a, mR-29a and miR-100) specifically regulated by HR-HPV E6 and E7 oncoproteins. Based on their preliminary data, eight miRNAs including miR-16, miR-22, miR-25, miR-27a, mR-29a, miR-92a, miR-100 and miR-378) were selected for further investigation, to determine which of the two E6 and E7 oncoproteins are their modulators.

HR-HPV E7 oncoprotein had a stronger effect than HR-HPV E6 oncoprotein on the positive regulation of miR-25, miR-378 and miR-16, while both viral oncoproteins regulate a moderate overexpression of miR-92a. The role of mir-25 in cervical cancer is assigned to invasion and metastasis by negatively regulation of RECK gene [77], while miR-16 by its CCNE1 target is involved in modulation of cell cycle progression [78].

Although miR-378 was associated with cervical cancer, its precise role has not yet been specified. Mir-92a promotes cell proliferation and cell migration as well as apoptosis blocking by down-regulation of PTEN [79]. The last four miRNAs investigated (miR-22, miR-27a, miR-29a and miR-100) were down-regulated by both E6 and E7 viral oncoproteins. While miR-22 inhibits tumor growth through a pro-apoptotic effect by targeting ATP citrate lyase [80], down-regulation of miR-27a led to overexpression of B4GALT3 that mediates malignancies of cervical cancer by β1-integrin pathway [81].

Cervical cancer progression is also mediated by the down-regulation of miR-29a resulting in HSP47 overexpression, which contributes to migration and invasion of cervical cancer [82], while down-regulation of miR-100 activates PLK1, increasing cell proliferation [83]. A common target of both E6 and E7 viral oncoproteins is miR-129, with tumor suppressor activity. In cervical cancer, miR-129 leads to up-regulation of CDK6 and therefore to increasing cell proliferation by G1-S cell cycle progression [84]. An important oncomir modulated by either E6 or E7 is miR-155, found to have high expression, and also associated with poor prognosis in cervical cancers [40]. MiR-155 is involved in proliferation of cervical tumor cells by down-regulation of LKB1 tumor suppressor gene [85]. Recent evidence demonstrates that not only HR-HPV E6 and E7 modulate the miRNAs expression in cervical cancer, but also HR-HPV E5 oncoprotein is involved in miRNAs targeting in cervical tumors. In a recent study, Liu et al. [86] demonstrated that E5 viral oncoprotein can target and down-regulate miR-196a, leading to increasing proliferation and cell growth by expression of HOXB8 and reduce apoptosis by modulating the caspase 3/7. In another study, Greco et al. [87] showed that in HaCaT human keratinocytes transfected with HPV 16 E5 (HaCaT-E5), the E5 oncoprotein can down-regulate miR-324-5p and miR203 and can up-regulate miR-146a. While miR-146 is involved in negative regulation of immune response in cervical cancer by targeting IRAK1 and TRAF6, miR-324-5p represents a negative modulator of the oncogenic Hedgehog pathway, contributing by its down-regulation leading to carcinogenesis and progression of cervical cancer. As we presented above, miR-203 is also targeted by E7 viral oncoprotein, being involved in epithelial cell differentiation and tumor progression [75].

4. MiRNAs expression in pre-neoplasic lesions and cervical cancer

Similar to other cancers, miRNA profiling in cervical cancer tissues was a topic intensively studied. Different studies involving different designs, from comparing normal and cancer tissues, primary and metastatic lesions, samples collected before and after surgery or therapy reported distinct miRNA profiles in cervical cancer.

There were studies, which used cervical cancer tissue and normal tissue samples from adjacent spots. The normal tissues were harvested from spots located 2–5 cm beyond the boundary of the tumor of the same individual or from healthy individuals. Therefore, the cervical cancer samples and the normal tissue samples were very likely to have similar histological structures. Patients that were enrolled in these studies had not received chemo- or radiotherapy prior to sample collection, which in most cases, occurred during surgery. In this regard, Rao et al. [88] determined miRNA profiling of 26 matched cervical cancer and normal tissue samples collected from 13 patients. MiRNA gene expression of cervical cancer tissues and normal adjacent tissues was assessed using CaptialBio mammalian miRNA array V3.0 (CapitalBio, Beijing, China). Microarray data analysis revealed that 18 miRNAs were significantly up-regulated and 19 miRNAs were significantly down-regulated in cervical cancer tissue when compared to normal tissue (**Table 2**). Significant analysis of microarray (SAM) using false discovery rate (FDR) showed that the expression levels of the microRNAs identified in this study were not dependent on lymph node metastasis (FDR = 0.529), vascular invasion (FDR = 0.371), or pathological differentiation (FDR = 0.163).

Author	Up-regulated miRNAs	Down-regulated miRNAs	Samples/cell lines	Method	Ref.
Rao et al.	miR-7, miR-429, miR-141, miR-142-5p, miR-31, miR-200a, miR-224, miR-20b, miR-18a, miR-200b, miR-93, miR-146b, miR-200c, rno-miR-93, miR-210, miR-20a; PREDICTED_MIR189, rno-miR-31, rno-miR-93	miR-127, rno-miR-140, miR-376a, miR-214, miR-218, miR-1, miR-368, miR-145, miR-100, miR-99a, miR-195, miR-320, miR-152, miR-497, miR-143, miR-99b, miR-10b, rno-miR-10b, mmu-miR-140	13 CC tissues/13 pair normal tissues	Microarray	[88]
Shen et al.	miR-224	–	126 CC/126 pair normal tissues	qRT-PCR	[89]
Lui et al.	miR-21	let-7b, let-7c, miR-23b, miR-196b, miR-143	Six cervical cell lines and 5 normal cervical tissues	Sequencing, Northern Blot	[90]
Han et al.	miR-21	–	30 CC tumor/30 normal tissue	qRT-PCR	[91]
Ding et al.	miR-657, miR-490-5p, miR-323-3p	miR-126, miR-96, miR-144	4 CC, PLN+/6 CC, PLN-	Microarray qRT-PCR	[92]
Cheung et al.	miR-518a, miR-34b, miR-34c, miR-20b, miR-338, miR-9, miR-512-5p, miR-424, miR-345, miR-10a	miR-193b, miR-203	24 CIN/9 healthy controls; validation 24 CIN; cross validation 51 CC	qRT-PCR	[93]

Author	Up-regulated miRNAs	Down-regulated miRNAs	Samples/cell lines	Method	Ref.
Ruiz et al.	miR-196a, miR-18b, miR-183, miR-500, miR-18a, miR-25, miR-182, miR-20b, miR-106a, miR-20a	miR-125b, miR-10b, miR-143, miR-337-5p, miR-199a-5p, miR-199b-3p, miR-127-3p, miR-214, miR-379, miR-145	4 CC/4 healthy controls and 12 tumoral cervical cell lines	Microarray	[94]
Pereira et al.	miR-148a, miR-302b, miR-10a, miR-196a, miR-132	miR-26a, miR-29a, miR-99a, miR-143, miR-145, miR-199a miR-203, miR-513	19 normal tissue, 4 squamous CC, 5 HSIL, 9 LSIL	Microarray, qRT-PCR	[95]
Li et al.	miR-155, miR-92a	mir-29a, miR-375, miR-195, mir-99a	51 CC, 51 CIN2/3, 21HR-HPV infected normal cervix, 49 normal specimens	Microarray, qRT-PCR	[96]

Abreviations: CC, cervical cancer; CIN, cervical intraepithelial neoplasia; HSIL, high-grade squamous intraepithelial lesion; LSIL, low-grade squamous intraepithelial lesion.

Table 2. MiRNAs expression in cervical cancer/CIN compared with normal tissues.

Another comparative study on cervical cancer and normal tissue was performed by Shen's group [89]. The qRT-PCR results showed a higher expression of miR-224. Moreover, miR-224 was significantly higher in advanced cervical cancers compared with early cervical cancers ($p = 0.02$) as well as in lymph node of metastatic-positive patients compared with lymph node metastatic-negative patients positive ($p = 0.008$), suggesting its role in cervical cancer progression. Furthermore, miR-224 was associated with less differentiated tumors ($p = 0.03$) and vascular invasion ($p = 0.01$), being proposed as an independent prognostic marker of cervical cancer.

Lui et al. [90] adopted a sequencing approach to identify new miRNAs in six human cervical cancer cell lines when compared with five normal cervical tissues. Their results revealed six miRNAs statistically significantly expressed in cervical tumor cell lines compared to normal cervix (**Table 2**). Five out from these miRNAs, such as let-7b, let-7c, miR-23b, miR-196b and miR-143, were down-regulated, while miR-21 was up-regulated in cervical tumor cells. MiR-21 and miR-143 were cross-validated in a new set of 29 pairs of cervical cancers and their matched normal tissues. Both these miRNAs have confirmed higher, respectively, lower expressions when compared to normal cervical tissue, qualifying them as markers for cervical cancer.

Another approach was to assess single miRNAs in cervical cancer tissue samples as biomarkers for diagnosis, and prognostic. In line with this view, Han et al. [91] compared the expression levels of miR-21 in 30 pairs of cervical cancer and normal tissue samples. Cervical tumor samples and normal tissue were collected from the same patients. The normal tissues were harvested beyond a 5 cm borderline from the tumor, in order to ensure the structure similarity between the tissue samples. MiR-21 quantification by qRT-PCR showed a higher expression level in cervical cancer tissues than in the normal ones with an average fold change of 4.02 and

p value <0.05. Moreover, miR-21 up-regulation was correlated with HPV16 infection by a relative expression level of 2.37 in HPV16 positive cases and only 1.94 in HPV16 negative cases. MiR-21 activity was also correlated with clinicopathological parameters including depth of invasion $p = 0.031$ and lymph node metastasis $p = 0.015$.

Ding et al. [92] reported a miR-microarray analysis where they identified a specific miRNA profile for metastatic cancers (PLN-positive) compared with non-metastatic cases (PLN-negative). Thirty-nine miRNAs with FC > 4 were included in this molecular signature; 22 miRNAs were significantly up-regulated, and 17 miRNAs were significantly down-regulated in the PLN-positive group when compared with PLN-negative group (**Table 2**). Six of these miRNAs including miR-126, miR-96, miR-144, miR-657, miR-490-5p and miR-323-3p for which were identified tumor associated putative target genes, involved in cell proliferation, apoptosis, tumor invasion and metastasis, were validated by qRT-PCR. However, they suggested that their data have to be confirmed on larger studies before making a reliable hypothesis related to these miRNAs.

Another important approach was to identify miRNAs for early diagnosis of cervical cancer. Cheung et al. [93] tried to identify a specific miRNA signature for CIN and to reveal what miRNAs could be involved in cervical carcinogenesis. Twenty-four high-grade cervical intraepithelial carcinoma (CIN 2/3) and nine normal cervical epithelium samples were used in a testing study for miRNA profiling, using qRT-PCR method for screening the expression of 202 target miRNAs. The obtained results, a set of 12 miRNAs (**Table 2**) statistically significantly expressed (FC ≥ 2, $p < 0.05$) between CIN and normal tissue, were further validated in a validation set of 24 high-grade CIN samples. Because permutation analysis returned 0.0% FDR for this set of miRNAs, a new analysis on an independent cohort of 51 squamous cell carcinomas was proposed, to reveal the miRNAs associated with cervical carcinogenesis. The fold change values of up-regulated miRNAs between CIN patients and normal subjects were ranging between 2.07 and 3.53 and between 2.67 and 2.81 for down-regulated ones. In the case of squamous cell carcinoma (SCC), seven miRNAs of 12 validated for CIN samples were identified as important for cancer progression. From these, miR-9, miR-20b, miR-345, miR-338, miR-518a and miR-512-5p were up-regulated, and miR-203 was down-regulated in cervical cancers versus normal epithelium control. Consequently, a specific miRNA signature that can distinguish CIN and cervical tumors from normal cervical epithelium was proposed. In the same line, Ruiz's group [94] used a microarray approach to identify differentially expressed miRNAs in cervical cancer cell lines as well as in cervical cancer and normal tissues. They studied miRNA expression on 12 cervical cancer cell lines, four cervical cancer tumor tissues and four normal tissue samples. They identified a set of miRNAs with significantly abnormal expression, of which, miR-196a had the highest expression level for cervical cancer tissues ($p = 4.75E{-}04$) and cancer cell lines ($p = 1.32E{-}07$). Up-regulation of miR-196a was confirmed by qRT-PCR analysis in cervical cancer tissues, low-grade squamous intraepithelial lesion (LSIL) and high-grade squamous intraepithelial lesion (HSIL) and cervical cancer cell lines. A highest up-regulation of miR-196a was observed in cervical cancer cell lines and a slight up-regulation in cervical cancer tissues. Other 19 miRNAs were found statistically significantly expressed in microarray analysis; nine of them were up-regulated, while the rest of 10 were down-regulated (**Table 2**).

Pereira et al. [95] profiled miRNA expression in a heterogenous set of 25 cervical tissues including 19 normal cervical tissue, four squamous cervical carcinoma, five high-grade squamous intraepithelial lesions (HSILs) and nine low-grade squamous intraepithelial lesions (LSILs). MiRNA profiling revealed a high variability of their expression among normal samples and a lack of clear separation of normal, pre-neoplasic and cervical cancer samples. One of the reasons claimed by authors was related to the fact that a part of normal cervical epitheliums harvested from area adjacent to the tumors were HPV infected. However, they identified two sets of statistically up-regulated and down-regulated miRNAs between precancerous and cancerous samples when compared with normal cervical tissues. Eight down-regulated miRNAs including miR-26a, miR-29a, miR-99a, miR-143, miR-145, miR-199a miR-203, miR-513 and five overexpressed miRNAs including miR-148a, miR-302b, miR-10a, miR-196a and miR-132 were associated with transition from normal cervix to both precancerous stages (atypical dysplasia) and cancer.

Ly et al. [96] profiled miRNA-microarray expression in six HPV16-positive cervical cancers, six HPV16-positive intraepithelial neopasia (CIN2/3) and six normal cervix tissues. They identified a set of 31 statistically significant miRNAs that distinguish cervical tumors from precancerous and normal samples. Six miRNAs (miR-155, miR-92a mir-29a, miR-375, miR-195 and miR-99a) were further successfully validated in a panel of 91 samples including 24 HPV16-positive cervical cancers, 24 HPV 16-positive CIN2/3 and 43 normal cervical tissues. Considering that cervical cells can be infected by different HR-HPV not only by HPV16, they also investigated and validated the expression of these six miRNAs in a larger group of 45 HR-HPV + cervical cancer, 45 HR-HPV + CIN2/3 and 43 normal cervical tissues.

5. MiRNAs expression in serum of patients with pre-neoplasic lesions and cervical cancer

Due to their high stability in easy accessible body fluids and their proved differential expression between cervical cancer and normal tissue, miRNAs have arisen as potential biomarkers for diagnosis and prediction of this disease.

In this regards, Jia et al. [97] performed a sequencing experiment to identify specific miRNAs in the serum of cervical cancer patients and normal subjects. They identified a set of 12 miRNAs differentially expressed between two groups. Cross-validation on a second set of 103 patients and 74 controls confirmed the significant up-regulation of five microRNAs (miR-21, mIR-29a, miR-200a, miR-25 and miR-486-5p) in cervical cancer when compared to the negative controls. MiR-21, one of the highest up-regulated microRNAs, was previously reported as overexpressed in cervical tumors, being an oncomir associated with poor prognosis [90, 91]. The diagnostic value of selected miRNAs was assessed by ROC analysis, showing that with each subsequent miR addition, the biomarker panel gained a higher sensitivity and specificity in discriminating cervical cancer from controls. With an AUC value of 0.908 (95% CI: 0.868–0.948), these results suggest the potential of the five microRNAs as noninvasive markers in cervical cancer.

Serum miRNAs could become valuable prognostic biomarkers (**Table 3**), aiding clinicians in treatment decision, to distinguish between cases that could be treated by using the classic therapy and the ones that might need a different approach because of a higher risk of developing lymph node metastasis.

Author	Serum microRNAs	Cases	Technology	Validation/cross validation	Test accuracy	Ref.
Jia et al.	↑miR-21 ↑miR-29a ↑miR-200a ↑miR-25 ↑miR-486-5p	213 CC patients 158 controls	Solexa sequencing qRT-PCR	103 patients 74 controls	CC vs. healthy AUC 0.908; 95% CI: 0.868-0.948; sensitivity: 81.0%, specificity 88.6%	[97]
Chen et al.	↑miR-205	60 CC patients60 controls	qRT-PCR	Same subjects 60 CC60 controls	LN+ vs LN− 0.694; sensitivity: 71.1%, specificity: 72.7% moderately differentiated vs poorly differetiated 0.717; sensitivity: 76.5%, a specificity: 73.1%	[98]
Zhao et al.	↑miR-1246 ↑miR-20a ↑miR-2392 ↑miR-3147 ↑miR-3162-5p ↑miR-4484	40 CC LN+ 40 CC LN− 20 controls	Microarray qRT-PCR	–	LN+ vs LN− AUC 0.932; 95% CI: 0.884-0.980, sensitivity 0.856, specificity 0.850	[99]
Ma et al.	↑miR-20a ↑miR-203	40 CC LN+ 40 CC LN− 20 controls	qRT-PCR	–	miR-20a LN+ vs LN− AUC 0.734; 95% CI: 1.137–2.118, sensitivity: 75%, specificity: 72.5% miR-203 LN+ vsLN− AUC 0.658; sensitivity: 65%, specificity: 62.5%	[100]
Yu et al.	↓miR-218	90 CC 50 controls	qRT-PCR	–	cc vs normal expression levels 1.000 vs 0.392 LN+ vs LN− expression levels 0.235 vs 0.468	[101]
Zhang et al.	↑miR-16-2 ↑miR-497 ↑miR-2861 ↓miR-195	184 CC patients 186 CIN 193 controls	qRT-PCR	85 CC 91 CIN 93 controls	CC vs healthy AUC 0.849; 95% CI: 0.813–0.886; sensitivity: 73.1%, specificity: 88.4% CC vs CIN AUC 0.829; 95% CI: 0.794–0.865; sensitivity: 71.4%, specificity: 67.2% cin vs healthy AUC 0.734; 95% CI, 0.683-0.784; sensitivity: 62.6%, specificity: 88.9%	[102]

Author	Serum microRNAs	Cases	Technology	Validation/cross validation	Test accuracy	Ref.
Nagamitsu et al.	↑miR-1920	70 CC patients 55 CIN 31 controls	Microarray qRT-PCR	45 CC patients 55 CIN 31 controls	CC vs healthy0.7957; 95% CI: 0.6937-0.8977; sensitivity: 90.3%, specificity: 62.2%,	[103]
Liu et al.	↑miR-196a	105 CC patients 86 CIN 50 controls	qRT-PCR	–	–	[104]

Abbreviations: CC, cervical cancer; CIN, cervical intraepithelial neoplasia; LN+, lymph node positive; LN−, lymph node negative; AUC, area under curve.

Table 3. MiRNAs expression in serum serum of patients with pre-neoplasic lesions and cervical cancer.

Using microarrays screening tools, Chen et al. [98] identified 89 miRNAs that had different expressions both in serum and in tissue samples of positive lymph node metastasis cervical cancer patients when compared to healthy controls. For further analysis, they restricted the number of microRNAs of interest, by choosing the microRNAs with the highest expression levels that are presented in both serum and tissue samples. They identified a six-miRNA panel (miR-1246, miR-20a, miR-2392, miR-3147, miR-3162-5p and miR-4484) with a diagnostic value for lymph node metastasis in cervical cancer patients, having a sensitivity of 0.856 and a specificity of 0.850.

Consistent cervical cancer serum levels of miR-20a were reported by Zhao et al. [99]. miR-20a being significantly up-regulated in serum samples collected from females with cervical cancer stages I–IIA, when compared to healthy donors. Moreover, higher differences were reported in serum samples from patients with positive lymph node metastasis (LN+) than in the ones without lymph node metastasis (LN−). They showed that miR-20a expression level could be used as a lymph node metastasis diagnosis tool, distinguishing LN+ from LN− patients with a moderate accuracy (AUC = 0.734) the test having a sensitivity of 75%, and a specificity of 72.5%. They also measured the expression level of miR-203 in serum samples of cervical cancer patients and healthy donors. Although it was observed a significant up-regulation of serum miR-203 in cervical cancer patients, miR-203 showed a low accuracy for distinguishing LN+ from LN− patients.

Ma's group [100] measured miR-205 level in blood and tissue samples of cervical cancer patients and paired healthy controls. They found a fivefold up-regulation of miR-205 in serum from cervical cancer patients, comparing to normal, and threefold up-regulation in tissue samples. Moreover, a higher expression level of miR-205 was correlated with an advanced cancer stage, a worse overall survival rate, and metastasis. As a prognosis biomarker, miR-205 expression level could differentiate between metastatic and non-metastatic cases with a sensitivity of 71.1% and specificity of 72.7%, and distinguish poorly differentiated tumors from that moderately differentiated ones with a sensitivity of 76.5% and a specificity of 73.1%.

Yu's group [101] investigated if serum miR-218 can be associated with cervical cancer. Accordingly, they identified reduced level of miR-218 in serum samples of 90 cervical cancer patients (expression level 0.392 ± 0.021) when compared to 50 healthy controls (expression level 1.000 ± 0.062). Quantitative RT-PCR showed even more decreasing levels of miR-218 in cervical cancer patients with advanced stages (0.128 ± 0.016) compared to earlier ones (0.425 ± 0.033). Moreover, they observed the same tendency for those patients presenting lymph node metastasis (0.235 ± 0.020) compared to non-metastatic cases (0.468 ± 0.018), and it suggested that miR-218 could represent a marker for prognosis. An interesting observation was that miR-218 expression level was lower for adenocarcinoma (0.216 ± 0.016) than for squamous cell cervical cancer (0.399 ± 0.019).

Timely biomarker detection would be of a great importance, considering the increased chances of survival and lower recurrence rates at early stages. Also, a blood-based biomarker that has a comparable or higher sensitivity and specificity than Pap test would be of a great benefit especially in the areas where high-quality medical care and screening are not available.

In line with this view, Zhang et al. [102] performed a qRT-PCR-based screening study evaluating the performance of circulating miRNAs as diagnostic biomarkers in the serum of patients with cervical cancer and patients with CIN. The study followed a multi-step approach: screening, testing and validation. For validation, they used randomly selected cervical cancer patients, CIN subjects and healthy individuals as negative controls. MirRNAs identified in the first cohort of patients in the screening step were tested in a second cohort and finally cross-validated on a third group of patients. A panel of four miRNAs (miR-16-2, miR-497, miR-2861, miR-195) with significantly aberrant expression was selected to discriminate cervical cancer from healthy subjects (AUC: 0.849; 95% CI: 0.813–0.886; sensitivity: 73.1%, specificity: 88.4%) and CIN (AUC: 0.829; 95% CI: 0.794–0.865; sensitivity: 71.4%, specificity: 67.2%). This 4-miRNA signature also distinguishes CIN from healthy subjects (AUC: 0.734; 95% CI: 0.683–0.784; sensitivity: 62.6%, specificity: 88.9%).

Following a similar workflow, Nagamitsu et al. [103] reported a recent microarray study that identified a panel of four up-regulated miRNAs (miR-485-5p, miR-1246, miR-1275, miR-1290) in the serum of cervical cancer patients. Mir-1290 was particularly up-regulated, so the group further investigated its expression level in the sera of CIN individuals and cervical cancer patients at different stages. The results showed that miR-1290 levels could differentiate cervical cancer patients from healthy subjects with an AUC value of 0.7957 (95% CI: 0.6937–0.8977; sensitivity: 90.3%; specificity: 62.2%). Also, miR-1290 up-regulation was correlated with cancer progression, with lowest expression in the control group and gradually increased expression from CIN2 to locally advanced cervical cancers, showing biomarker potential for cervical cancer diagnosis in early stages.

In another study, Liu's group [104] evaluated the expression of serum miR-196a in 105 cervical cancer patients, 85 CIN individuals and 50 healthy subjects. Their data revealed a significantly higher relative expression level of miR-196a in cervical cancer patients than in both healthy and CIN individuals, and higher expression in CIN than in healthy subjects. The study aimed to identify the clinical significance of serum miR-196a in cervical cancer and CIN patients. Their results showed an association between miR-196a and clinical parameters of cervical cancer patients, such as tumor size, lymph node (LN) metastasis, FIGO stage and cancer grade, but no association with HPV infection, age, or cell type. Also, they observed different levels of miR-196a expression depending on CIN grade, with a lower expression in CINI and CINII and a significantly higher expression level in CINIII. Moreover, overall survival of cervical cancer patients was negatively correlated with higher miR-196a expression. These results suggest that serum miR-196a could represent a reliable biomarker for early diagnosis and prognosis of cervical cancer.

6. MiRNAs expression in exfoliated cells of cervix

In addition to cervical cancer screening tests by using serum-based diagnosis biomarkers, in a recent study, Tian et al. [105] have approached a new screening method for early detection of cervical cancer. This group collected residual exfoliated cell samples from HPV-positive subjects that underwent Pap test. Samples were triaged by Pap test and colposcopy in six groups, depending on the lesions grade, ranging from normal to ASCUS, LSIL, ASC-H, HSIL, and finally CC. Sampled cells from 1021 HPV-positive women were used for measuring the expression levels of several microRNAs, which were previously detected as abnormally regulated in cervical cancer (miR-424/miR-375/miR-34a/miR-218/miR-92a/miR-93). Detailed cytological examination classified the subjects by CIN grade. Quantitative RT-PCR analysis showed that relative expression levels of miR-218, miR-34a, miR-424 and miR-375 were significantly lower in more advanced CIN grades (CIN2+ and CIN3+) than in the incipient ones (CIN-1 and CIN-2), suggesting that those microRNAs could be used as candidate biomarkers in cervical cancer screening. For determining the diagnosis value, the group performed ROC analysis for miR-424, miR-375, miR-34a and miR-218 and compared them to the ROC curve for Pap test. Both miR-424 and miR-375 detection in cervical exfoliated cells had a greater AUC (0.828 for miR-424 and 0.760 for miR-375) and a higher sensitivity (82.3% for miR-424 and 80.9% for miR-375, respectively) and specificity (70% for miR-424 and 71.2% for miR-375, respectively) in identifying high-grade CIN (CIN3+) than Pap test (AUC: 0.699; sensitivity 69.8%, specificity 70%). A lower performance was registered for miR-34 and miR-218. In conclusion, this study opens future challenges in non-invasive diagnosis procedures. MicroRNA detection in cervical exfoliated cells could be an effective option for triage of HPV-positive women and incipient cancer detection, especially for those areas where well-trained cytologists are lacking.

7. MiRNAs modulate treatment response in cervical cancer

The molecular mechanisms of resistance to radiation in cervical cancer are not well understood. The discovery of miRNAs opened the opportunity to research for new molecules that mediate treatment response, with potential to be developed into new targeting strategies and/or prediction algorithms in cervical cancer treatment. However, the current knowledge is still limited, and there are just a few reports describing the role of miRNAs as modulators of treatment response in cervical cancer.

In a recent study, Song et al. [106] investigated the role of miR-375 in radiotherapy resistance in HR-HPV-positive cervical cancers. They evaluated tissue and serum expression of miR-375 in both cervical cancer patients ($n = 22$) and healthy control subjects ($n = 20$) highlighting significantly down-regulated expression also in tissue ($p < 0.001$) and serum ($p < 0.001$) of cancer patients when compared to normal individuals. The authors also assessed the miR-375 expression level in serum and tissue samples at 6 months after completion of the radiotherapy treatment and correlated its expression with clinical and histological data. Their data showed low expression of miR-375 in tissue ($p < 0.001$) and serum ($p < 0.001$) of radioresistant patients when compared with radiosensitive patients. Further investigations have proved that miR-375 may induce radioresistance in cervical cancer cells by targeting UBE3A and BIRC5 (surviving) and regulate apoptosis through the 53 pathway.

Ye et al. [107] reported decreased miR-145 expression in tumors and cervical cell lines when compared with cervical non-tumor tissue and normal cell lines. Five potential targets of miR-145 including HLTF, CUT2, BCR, BUFIP2 and ZCH11A were identified by in silico analysis, but only HLTFs were further investigated due to its mRNA highest expression (1.96-fold). The expression of HLTF was higher in cervical tumors than in normal tissues and significantly negatively correlated with miR-145 in cervical cancers. Moreover, performing luciferase reporting assay, this group has proved that HTLF is a specific target of miR-145. HTLF influences the outcome of radiotherapy in cervical tumors playing an important role in chromatin remodeling and enhancing DNA damage repair capacity of cervical tumor cells, therefore miR-145 down-regulation could lead to radioresistance in cervical cancers.

Ke et al. [108] investigated the role of miR-181a in radiotherapy resistance of cervical cancers. MiRNA microarray profiling in seven radio-resistant cervical samples and 11 radio-sensitive cervical tumors led to the identification of eight miRNAs (miR-181a, miR-21, miR-30, miR-23a, miR-16-2, miR-378, miR-18a and miR-221) significantly expressed between groups. Further investigation showed that miR-181a has no effect on cell proliferation but lead to inhibition of apoptosis by targeting the PRKCD gene and decreasing the caspase 3/7 activity. The authors suggested that miR-181a protects cervical tumor cells from radiation-inducing death by inhibiting of apoptosis.

8. Conclusion

Data presented above provide evidences that miRNAs modulated by HR-HPV E5, E6 and E7 oncoproteins could be investigated as potential biomarkers for early diagnosis of pre-neoplasic and neoplasic lesions of the cervix. Moreover, miRNAs identified in serum and exfoliated cervical cells could be taken into account as valuable minimal invasive markers for monitoring cervical cancer progression and its treatment response.

Acknowledgements

The work for this chapter was supported by the UEFISCDI Program-PNII-PT-PCCA-2011-3.2-1328 (Grant 96/2012).

http://dx.doi.org/10.5772/68011

Author details

Ovidiu Balacescu[1]*, Loredana Balacescu[1], Oana Baldasici[1], Oana Tudoran[1] and Patriciu Achimas-Cadariu[2]

*Address all correspondence to: ovidiubalacescu@iocn.ro

1 Department of Functional Genomics, Proteomics and Experimental Pathology, The Oncology Institute, Cluj-Napoca, Romania

2 Department of Surgical and Gynecological Oncology, University of Medicine and Pharmacy, Cluj-Napoca, Romania and Department of Surgery, The Oncology Institute, Cluj-Napoca, Romania

References

[1] American Cancer Society. Global Cancer Facts & Figures 3rd Edition. Atlanta: American Cancer Society; 2015 **2**:34-36

[2] Goldie SJ, Gaffikin L, Goldhaber-Fiebert JD, Gordillo-Tobar A, Levin C, Mahe C, et al. Cost-effectiveness of cervical-cancer screening in five developing countries. N Engl J Med. 2005 **353**:2158-68.

[3] Colombo N, Carinelli S, Colombo A, Marini C, Rollo D, Sessa C. Cervical cancer: ESMO Clinical Practice Guidelines for diagnosis, treatment and follow-up. Ann Oncol. 2012 **23 Suppl 7**:vii27-32.

[4] Ambros V. The evolution of our thinking about microRNAs. Nat Med. 2008 **14**:1036-40.

[5] Hrdlickova B, de Almeida RC, Borek Z, Withoff S. Genetic variation in the non-coding genome: Involvement of micro-RNAs and long non-coding RNAs in disease. Biochim Biophys Acta. 2014 **1842**:1910-22.

[6] Lewis BP, Burge CB, Bartel DP. Conserved seed pairing, often flanked by adenosines, indicates that thousands of human genes are microRNA targets. Cell. 2005 **120**:15-20.

[7] Lim LP, Lau NC, Garrett-Engele P, Grimson A, Schelter JM, Castle J, et al. Microarray analysis shows that some microRNAs downregulate large numbers of target mRNAs. Nature. 2005 **433**:769-73.

[8] Krek A, Grun D, Poy MN, Wolf R, Rosenberg L, Epstein EJ, et al. Combinatorial microRNA target predictions. Nat Genet. 2005 **37**:495-500.

[9] Croce CM. Causes and consequences of microRNA dysregulation in cancer. Nat Rev Genet. 2009 **10**:704-14.

[10] Lopez-Serra P, Esteller M. DNA methylation-associated silencing of tumor-suppressor microRNAs in cancer. Oncogene. 2012 **31**:1609-22.

[11] Calin GA, Dumitru CD, Shimizu M, Bichi R, Zupo S, Noch E, et al. Frequent deletions and down-regulation of micro-RNA genes miR15 and miR16 at 13q14 in chronic lymphocytic leukemia. Proc Natl Acad Sci U S A. 2002 **99**:15524-9.

[12] Calin GA, Sevignani C, Dumitru CD, Hyslop T, Noch E, Yendamuri S, et al. Human microRNA genes are frequently located at fragile sites and genomic regions involved in cancers. Proc Natl Acad Sci U S A. 2004 **101**:2999-3004.

[13] Calin GA, Liu CG, Sevignani C, Ferracin M, Felli N, Dumitru CD, et al. MicroRNA profiling reveals distinct signatures in B cell chronic lymphocytic leukemias. Proc Natl Acad Sci U S A. 2004 **101**:11755-60.

[14] Griffiths-Jones S. The microRNA Registry. Nucleic Acids Res. 2004 **32**:D109-11.

[15] Lander ES, Linton LM, Birren B, Nusbaum C, Zody MC, Baldwin J, et al. Initial sequencing and analysis of the human genome. Nature. 2001 **409**:860-921.

[16] Pennisi E. Genomics. ENCODE project writes eulogy for junk DNA. Science. 2012 **337**:1159, 61.

[17] Kim VN, Han J, Siomi MC. Biogenesis of small RNAs in animals. Nat Rev Mol Cell Biol. 2009 **10**:126-39.

[18] Lee Y, Kim M, Han J, Yeom KH, Lee S, Baek SH, et al. MicroRNA genes are transcribed by RNA polymerase II. EMBO J. 2004 **23**:4051-60.

[19] Borchert GM, Lanier W, Davidson BL. RNA polymerase III transcribes human microRNAs. Nat Struct Mol Biol. 2006 **13**:1097-101.

[20] Kim VN. MicroRNA biogenesis: coordinated cropping and dicing. Nat Rev Mol Cell Biol. 2005 **6**:376-85.

[21] Lund E, Guttinger S, Calado A, Dahlberg JE, Kutay U. Nuclear export of microRNA precursors. Science. 2004 **303**:95-8.

[22] Winter J, Jung S, Keller S, Gregory RI, Diederichs S. Many roads to maturity: microRNA biogenesis pathways and their regulation. Nat Cell Biol. 2009 **11**:228-34.

[23] Meister G. Argonaute proteins: functional insights and emerging roles. Nat Rev Genet. 2013 **14**:447-59.

[24] Robinson VL. Rethinking the central dogma: noncoding RNAs are biologically relevant. Urol Oncol. 2009 **27**:304-6.

[25] Cimmino A, Calin GA, Fabbri M, Iorio MV, Ferracin M, Shimizu M, et al. miR-15 and miR-16 induce apoptosis by targeting BCL2. Proc Natl Acad Sci U S A. 2005 **102**:13944-9.

[26] Lu J, Getz G, Miska EA, Alvarez-Saavedra E, Lamb J, Peck D, et al. MicroRNA expression profiles classify human cancers. Nature. 2005 **435**:834-8.

[27] He L, Thomson JM, Hemann MT, Hernando-Monge E, Mu D, Goodson S, et al. A microRNA polycistron as a potential human oncogene. Nature. 2005 **435**:828-33.

[28] Mihailovich M, Bremang M, Spadotto V, Musiani D, Vitale E, Varano G, et al. miR-17-92 fine-tunes MYC expression and function to ensure optimal B cell lymphoma growth. Nat Commun. 2015 **6**:8725.

[29] O'Donnell KA, Wentzel EA, Zeller KI, Dang CV, Mendell JT. c-Myc-regulated microRNAs modulate E2F1 expression. Nature. 2005 **435**:839-43.

[30] Berindan-Neagoe I, Monroig Pdel C, Pasculli B, Calin GA. MicroRNAome genome: a treasure for cancer diagnosis and therapy. CA Cancer J Clin. 2014 **64**:311-36.

[31] Mar-Aguilar F, Rodriguez-Padilla C, Resendez-Perez D. Web-based tools for microRNAs involved in human cancer. Oncol Lett. 2016 **11**:3563-70.

[32] Willis RE. Human gene control by vital oncogenes: revisiting a theoretical model and its implications for targeted cancer therapy. Int J Mol Sci. 2012 **13**:316-35.

[33] Pfeffer SR, Yang CH, Pfeffer LM. The Role of miR-21 in Cancer. Drug Dev Res. 2015 **76**:270-7.

[34] Peralta-Zaragoza O, Deas J, Meneses-Acosta A, De la OGF, Fernandez-Tilapa G, Gomez-Ceron C, et al. Relevance of miR-21 in regulation of tumor suppressor gene PTEN in human cervical cancer cells. BMC Cancer. 2016 **16**:215.

[35] Zhang BG, Li JF, Yu BQ, Zhu ZG, Liu BY, Yan M. microRNA-21 promotes tumor proliferation and invasion in gastric cancer by targeting PTEN. Oncol Rep. 2012 **27**:1019-26.

[36] Liwak-Muir U, Dobson CC, Naing T, Wylie Q, Chehade L, Baird SD, et al. ERK8 is a novel HuR kinase that regulates tumour suppressor PDCD4 through a miR-21 dependent mechanism. Oncotarget. 2016 **7**:1439-50.

[37] Xue X, Liu Y, Wang Y, Meng M, Wang K, Zang X, et al. MiR-21 and MiR-155 promote non-small cell lung cancer progression by down regulating SOCS1, SOCS6, and PTEN. Oncotarget. 2016 **7**:84508-19.

[38] Willimott S, Wagner SD. miR-125b and miR-155 contribute to BCL2 repression and proliferation in response to CD40 ligand (CD154) in human leukemic B-cells. J Biol Chem. 2012 **287**:2608-17.

[39] Higgs G, Slack F. The multiple roles of microRNA-155 in oncogenesis. J Clin Bioinforma. 2013 **3**:17.

[40] Fang H, Shuang D, Yi Z, Sheng H, Liu Y. Up-regulated microRNA-155 expression is associated with poor prognosis in cervical cancer patients. Biomed Pharmacother. 2016 **83**:64-9.

[41] Garofalo M, Quintavalle C, Romano G, Croce CM, Condorelli G. miR221/222 in cancer: their role in tumor progression and response to therapy. Curr Mol Med. 2012 **12**:27-33.

[42] Felli N, Fontana L, Pelosi E, Botta R, Bonci D, Facchiano F, et al. MicroRNAs 221 and 222 inhibit normal erythropoiesis and erythroleukemic cell growth via kit receptor down-modulation. Proc Natl Acad Sci U S A. 2005 **102**:18081-6.

[43] Xiang J, Wu J. Feud or friend? The role of the miR-17-92 cluster in tumorigenesis. Curr Genomics. 2010 **11**:129-35.

[44] Fuziwara CS, Kimura ET. Insights into regulation of the miR-17-92 cluster of miRNAs in cancer. Front Med (Lausanne). 2015 **2**:64.

[45] Mestdagh P, Bostrom AK, Impens F, Fredlund E, Van Peer G, De Antonellis P, et al. The miR-17-92 microRNA cluster regulates multiple components of the TGF-beta pathway in neuroblastoma. Mol Cell. 2010 **40**:762-73.

[46] Hossain A, Kuo MT, Saunders GF. Mir-17-5p regulates breast cancer cell proliferation by inhibiting translation of AIB1 mRNA. Mol Cell Biol. 2006 **26**:8191-201.

[47] Bonci D, De Maria R. miR-15/miR-16 loss, miR-21 upregulation, or deregulation of their target genes predicts poor prognosis in prostate cancer patients. Mol Cell Oncol. 2016 **3**:e1109744.

[48] Mobarra N, Shafiee A, Rad SM, Tasharrofi N, Soufi-Zomorod M, Hafizi M, et al. Overexpression of microRNA-16 declines cellular growth, proliferation and induces apoptosis in human breast cancer cells. In Vitro Cell Dev Biol Anim. 2015 **51**:604-11.

[49] Gomez-Gomez Y, Organista-Nava J, Gariglio P. Deregulation of the miRNAs expression in cervical cancer: human papillomavirus implications. Biomed Res Int. 2013 **2013**:407052.

[50] Samuel N, Wilson G, Id Said B, Pan A, Deblois G, Fischer NW, et al. Transcriptome-wide characterization of the endogenous miR-34A-p53 tumor suppressor network. Oncotarget. 2016 **7**:49611-22.

[51] Si W, Li Y, Shao H, Hu R, Wang W, Zhang K, et al. MiR-34a Inhibits Breast Cancer Proliferation and Progression by Targeting Wnt1 in Wnt/beta-Catenin Signaling Pathway. Am J Med Sci. 2016 **352**:191-9.

[52] Chandrasekaran KS, Sathyanarayanan A, Karunagaran D. Downregulation of HMGB1 by miR-34a is sufficient to suppress proliferation, migration and invasion of human cervical and colorectal cancer cells. Tumour Biol. 2016 **37**:13155-66.

[53] Zheng F, Zhang J, Luo S, Yi J, Wang P, Zheng Q, et al. miR-143 is associated with proliferation and apoptosis involving ERK5 in HeLa cells. Oncol Lett. 2016 **12**:3021-7.

[54] Song T, Zhang X, Wang C, Wu Y, Dong J, Gao J, et al. Expression of miR-143 reduces growth and migration of human bladder carcinoma cells by targeting cyclooxygenase-2. Asian Pac J Cancer Prev. 2011 **12**:929-33.

[55] Zou C, Xu Q, Mao F, Li D, Bian C, Liu LZ, et al. MiR-145 inhibits tumor angiogenesis and growth by N-RAS and VEGF. Cell Cycle. 2012 **11**:2137-45.

[56] Zhang J, Guo H, Zhang H, Wang H, Qian G, Fan X, et al. Putative tumor suppressor miR-145 inhibits colon cancer cell growth by targeting oncogene Friend leukemia virus integration 1 gene. Cancer. 2011 **117**:86-95.

[57] Cui SY, Wang R, Chen LB. MicroRNA-145: a potent tumour suppressor that regulates multiple cellular pathways. J Cell Mol Med. 2014 **18**:1913-26.

[58] Bernard HU, Burk RD, Chen Z, van Doorslaer K, zur Hausen H, de Villiers EM. Classification of papillomaviruses (PVs) based on 189 PV types and proposal of taxonomic amendments. Virology. 2010 **401**:70-9.

[59] Doorbar J, Egawa N, Griffin H, Kranjec C, Murakami I. Human papillomavirus molecular biology and disease association. Rev Med Virol. 2015 **25 Suppl 1**:2-23.

[60] Bruni L, Diaz M, Castellsague X, Ferrer E, Bosch FX, de Sanjose S. Cervical human papillomavirus prevalence in 5 continents: meta-analysis of 1 million women with normal cytological findings. J Infect Dis. 2010 **202**:1789-99.

[61] Guan P, Howell-Jones R, Li N, Bruni L, de Sanjose S, Franceschi S, et al. Human papillomavirus types in 115, 789 HPV-positive women: a meta-analysis from cervical infection to cancer. Int J Cancer. 2012 **131**:2349-59.

[62] Liu W, Gao G, Hu X, Wang Y, Schwarz JK, Chen JJ, et al. Activation of miR-9 by human papillomavirus in cervical cancer. Oncotarget. 2014 **5**:11620-30.

[63] Au Yeung CL, Tsang TY, Yau PL, Kwok TT. Human papillomavirus type 16 E6 induces cervical cancer cell migration through the p53/microRNA-23b/urokinase-type plasminogen activator pathway. Oncogene. 2011 **30**:2401-10.

[64] Riethdorf L, Riethdorf S, Petersen S, Bauer M, Herbst H, Janicke F, et al. Urokinase gene expression indicates early invasive growth in squamous cell lesions of the uterine cervix. J Pathol. 1999 **189**:245-50.

[65] Raver-Shapira N, Marciano E, Meiri E, Spector Y, Rosenfeld N, Moskovits N, et al. Transcriptional activation of miR-34a contributes to p53-mediated apoptosis. Mol Cell. 2007 **26**:731-43.

[66] Wang X, Meyers C, Guo M, Zheng ZM. Upregulation of p18Ink4c expression by oncogenic HPV E6 via p53-miR-34a pathway. Int J Cancer. 2011 **129**:1362-72.

[67] Sun F, Fu H, Liu Q, Tie Y, Zhu J, Xing R, et al. Downregulation of CCND1 and CDK6 by miR-34a induces cell cycle arrest. FEBS Lett. 2008 **582**:1564-8.

[68] Li Y, Liu J, Yuan C, Cui B, Zou X, Qiao Y. High-risk human papillomavirus reduces the expression of microRNA-218 in women with cervical intraepithelial neoplasia. J Int Med Res. 2010 **38**:1730-6.

[69] Jiang Z, Song Q, Zeng R, Li J, Lin X, Chen X, et al. MicroRNA-218 inhibits EMT, migration and invasion by targeting SFMBT1 and DCUN1D1 in cervical cancer. Oncotarget. 2016 **7**:45622-36.

[70] Yuan W, Xiaoyun H, Haifeng Q, Jing L, Weixu H, Ruofan D, et al. MicroRNA-218 enhances the radiosensitivity of human cervical cancer via promoting radiation induced apoptosis. Int J Med Sci. 2014 **11**:691-6.

[71] Gonzalez SL, Stremlau M, He X, Basile JR, Munger K. Degradation of the retinoblastoma tumor suppressor by the human papillomavirus type 16 E7 oncoprotein is important for functional inactivation and is separable from proteasomal degradation of E7. J Virol. 2001 **75**:7583-91.

[72] Ofir M, Hacohen D, Ginsberg D. MiR-15 and miR-16 are direct transcriptional targets of E2F1 that limit E2F-induced proliferation by targeting cyclin E. Mol Cancer Res. 2011 **9**:440-7.

[73] Myklebust MP, Bruland O, Fluge O, Skarstein A, Balteskard L, Dahl O. MicroRNA-15b is induced with E2F-controlled genes in HPV-related cancer. Br J Cancer. 2011 **105**:1719-25.

[74] Cardeal LB, Boccardo E, Termini L, Rabachini T, Andreoli MA, di Loreto C, et al. HPV16 oncoproteins induce MMPs/RECK-TIMP-2 imbalance in primary keratinocytes: possible implications in cervical carcinogenesis. PLoS One. 2012 **7**:e33585.

[75] Yi R, Poy MN, Stoffel M, Fuchs E. A skin microRNA promotes differentiation by repressing 'stemness'. Nature. 2008 **452**:225-9.

[76] Wang X, Wang HK, Li Y, Hafner M, Banerjee NS, Tang S, et al. microRNAs are biomarkers of oncogenic human papillomavirus infections. Proc Natl Acad Sci U S A. 2014 **111**:4262-7.

[77] Qiu G, Fang B, Xin G, Wei Q, Yuan X, Wu D. [miR-25 promotes cell proliferation by targeting RECK in human cervical carcinoma HeLa cells]. Xi Bao Yu Fen Zi Mian Yi Xue Za Zhi. 2015 **31**:40-3.

[78] Zubillaga-Guerrero MI, Alarcon-Romero Ldel C, Illades-Aguiar B, Flores-Alfaro E, Bermudez-Morales VH, Deas J, et al. MicroRNA miR-16-1 regulates CCNE1 (cyclin E1) gene expression in human cervical cancer cells. Int J Clin Exp Med. 2015 **8**:15999-6006.

[79] Yu Y, Zhang Y, Zhang S. MicroRNA-92 regulates cervical tumorigenesis and its expression is upregulated by human papillomavirus-16 E6 in cervical cancer cells. Oncol Lett. 2013 **6**:468-74.

[80] Xin M, Qiao Z, Li J, Liu J, Song S, Zhao X, et al. miR-22 inhibits tumor growth and metastasis by targeting ATP citrate lyase: evidence in osteosarcoma, prostate cancer, cervical cancer and lung cancer. Oncotarget. 2016 **7**:44252-65.

[81] Sun Y, Yang X, Liu M, Tang H. B4GALT3 up-regulation by miR-27a contributes to the oncogenic activity in human cervical cancer cells. Cancer Lett. 2016 **375**:284-92.

[82] Yamamoto N, Kinoshita T, Nohata N, Yoshino H, Itesako T, Fujimura L, et al. Tumor-suppressive microRNA-29a inhibits cancer cell migration and invasion via targeting HSP47 in cervical squamous cell carcinoma. Int J Oncol. 2013 **43**:1855-63.

[83] Li BH, Zhou JS, Ye F, Cheng XD, Zhou CY, Lu WG, et al. Reduced miR-100 expression in cervical cancer and precursors and its carcinogenic effect through targeting PLK1 protein. Eur J Cancer. 2011 **47**:2166-74.

[84] Wu J, Qian J, Li C, Kwok L, Cheng F, Liu P, et al. miR-129 regulates cell proliferation by downregulating Cdk6 expression. Cell Cycle. 2010 **9**:1809-18.

[85] Lao G, Liu P, Wu Q, Zhang W, Liu Y, Yang L, et al. Mir-155 promotes cervical cancer cell proliferation through suppression of its target gene LKB1. Tumour Biol. 2014 **35**:11933-8.

[86] Liu C, Lin J, Li L, Zhang Y, Chen W, Cao Z, et al. HPV16 early gene E5 specifically reduces miRNA-196a in cervical cancer cells. Sci Rep. 2015 **5**:7653.

[87] Greco D, Kivi N, Qian K, Leivonen SK, Auvinen P, Auvinen E. Human papillomavirus 16 E5 modulates the expression of host microRNAs. PLoS One. 2011 **6**:e21646.

[88] Rao Q, Shen Q, Zhou H, Peng Y, Li J, Lin Z. Aberrant microRNA expression in human cervical carcinomas. Med Oncol. 2012 **29**:1242-8.

[89] Shen SN, Wang LF, Jia YF, Hao YQ, Zhang L, Wang H. Upregulation of microRNA-224 is associated with aggressive progression and poor prognosis in human cervical cancer. Diagn Pathol. 2013 **8**:69.

[90] Lui WO, Pourmand N, Patterson BK, Fire A. Patterns of known and novel small RNAs in human cervical cancer. Cancer Res. 2007 **67**:6031-43.

[91] Han Y, Xu GX, Lu H, Yu DH, Ren Y, Wang L, et al. Dysregulation of miRNA-21 and their potential as biomarkers for the diagnosis of cervical cancer. Int J Clin Exp Pathol. 2015 **8**:7131-9.

[92] Ding H, Wu YL, Wang YX, Zhu FF. Characterization of the microRNA expression profile of cervical squamous cell carcinoma metastases. Asian Pac J Cancer Prev. 2014 **15**:1675-9.

[93] Cheung TH, Man KN, Yu MY, Yim SF, Siu NS, Lo KW, et al. Dysregulated microRNAs in the pathogenesis and progression of cervical neoplasm. Cell Cycle. 2012 **11**:2876-84.

[94] Villegas-Ruiz V, Juarez-Mendez S, Perez-Gonzalez OA, Arreola H, Paniagua-Garcia L, Parra-Melquiadez M, et al. Heterogeneity of microRNAs expression in cervical cancer cells: over-expression of miR-196a. Int J Clin Exp Pathol. 2014 **7**:1389-401.

[95] Pereira PM, Marques JP, Soares AR, Carreto L, Santos MA. MicroRNA expression variability in human cervical tissues. PLoS One. 2010 **5**:e11780.

[96] Li Y, Wang F, Xu J, Ye F, Shen Y, Zhou J, et al. Progressive miRNA expression profiles in cervical carcinogenesis and identification of HPV-related target genes for miR-29. J Pathol. 2011 **224**:484-95.

[97] Jia W, Wu Y, Zhang Q, Gao GE, Zhang C, Xiang Y. Expression profile of circulating microRNAs as a promising fingerprint for cervical cancer diagnosis and monitoring. Mol Clin Oncol. 2015 **3**:851-8.

[98] Chen J, Yao D, Li Y, Chen H, He C, Ding N, et al. Serum microRNA expression levels can predict lymph node metastasis in patients with early-stage cervical squamous cell carcinoma. Int J Mol Med. 2013 **32**:557-67.

[99] Zhao S, Yao D, Chen J, Ding N. Circulating miRNA-20a and miRNA-203 for screening lymph node metastasis in early stage cervical cancer. Genet Test Mol Biomarkers. 2013 **17**:631-6.

[100] Ma Q, Wan G, Wang S, Yang W, Zhang J, Yao X. Serum microRNA-205 as a novel biomarker for cervical cancer patients. Cancer Cell Int. 2014 **14**:81.

[101] Yu J, Wang Y, Dong R, Huang X, Ding S, Qiu H. Circulating microRNA-218 was reduced in cervical cancer and correlated with tumor invasion. J Cancer Res Clin Oncol. 2012 **138**:671-4.

[102] Zhang Y, Zhang D, Wang F, Xu D, Guo Y, Cui W. Serum miRNAs panel (miR-16-2*, miR-195, miR-2861, miR-497) as novel non-invasive biomarkers for detection of cervical cancer. Sci Rep. 2015 **5**:17942.

[103] Nagamitsu Y, Nishi H, Sasaki T, Takaesu Y, Terauchi F, Isaka K. Profiling analysis of circulating microRNA expression in cervical cancer. Mol Clin Oncol. 2016 **5**:189-94.

[104] Liu P, Xin F, Ma CF. Clinical significance of serum miR-196a in cervical intraepithelial neoplasia and cervical cancer. Genet Mol Res. 2015 **14**:17995-8002.

[105] Tian Q, Li Y, Wang F, Xu J, Shen Y, Ye F, et al. MicroRNA detection in cervical exfoliated cells as a triage for human papillomavirus-positive women. J Natl Cancer Inst. 2014 **106**(9). doi: 10.1093/jnci/dju241

[106] Song L, Liu S, Zeng S, Zhang L, Li X. miR-375 Modulates Radiosensitivity of HR-HPV-Positive Cervical Cancer Cells by Targeting UBE3A through the p53 Pathway. Med Sci Monit. 2015 **21**:2210-7.

[107] Ye C, Sun NX, Ma Y, Zhao Q, Zhang Q, Xu C, et al. MicroRNA-145 contributes to enhancing radiosensitivity of cervical cancer cells. FEBS Lett. 2015 **589**:702-9.

[108] Ke G, Liang L, Yang JM, Huang X, Han D, Huang S, et al. MiR-181a confers resistance of cervical cancer to radiation therapy through targeting the pro-apoptotic PRKCD gene. Oncogene. 2013 **32**:3019-27.